AF478697

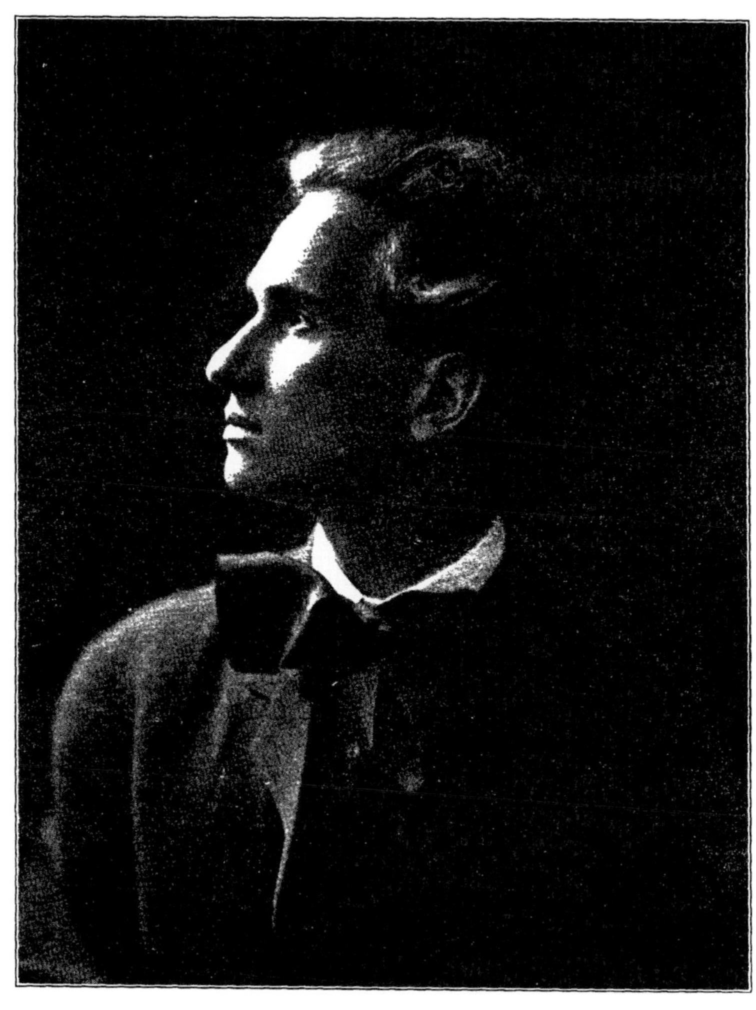

Yours in Truth and Love
Edward Earle Purinton

THE PHILOSOPHY

OF FASTING

A Message

for Sufferers and Sinners

BY

EDWARD EARLE PURINTON

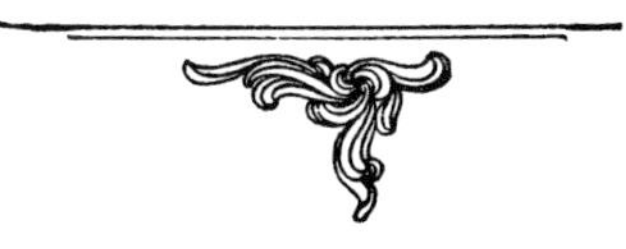

PUBLISHED BY

BENEDICT LUST

1906.

INDEX

THE PHILOSOPHY OF FASTING

A MESSAGE FOR SUFFERERS AND SINNERS

BY EDWARD EARLE PURINTON.

This book is the record of a soul's emancipation.

Only sufferers and sinners will understand it.

Because only sinners and sufferers are on the highway to Freedom.

The sinner *acts* without thinking—and is thereby made bold for better things.

The sufferer *feels* without thinking—and is thereby made receptive for finer things.

The reasoner *thinks* without either feeling or acting—and is thereby made too numb to suffer, too fearful to be aught but impotently virtuous.

Not to the brain of the worldly-wise, that dusty storehouse of race rubbish, will my message appeal. But to the heart of the sufferer softened through anguish, to the soul of the sinner strengthened through abandon, and to the spirit of the child quickened from its nearness to fairies and angels.

Such as are pitied, despised or condemned I call my brothers and sisters. Borne from the stagnant surface of being into the wild engulfment of its whirlpool soul, these have sounded the misery of the depths, have lain half-dead amid the wreckage on the shore, and are now able to appreciate and determined to attain the glory of the heights illumed by Truth.

Come, let us mount together. I have explored both the valley and the summit. And I promise you the way is plain.

Don't be needlessly apprehensive at the start—this isn't a missionary tract. Missionary literature is distributed by persons too good to touch the folks next-door. You see Asiatic heathen don't need fumigating so long as we proselyte them by post.

Now there are thousands of worthy people who honestly believe that their mission on earth is to reform, convert and reconstruct this world before sun-up to-morrow morning. Naturally they must write a book this afternoon, address at least one mass meeting this evening, and devote the feverishly fugitive midnight hours to personal exhortation. Even then a new dawn overtakes them. And the sun shamelessly smiles on a race still unredeemed.

These self-appointed leaders require devotees. Nothing but their following justifies their faith. And if their book isn't read, or their discourse applauded, they bemoan to themselves how signally they have failed.

How incomprehensible. Has not Truth all eternity wherein to speak to the souls of men? And if the message be true, it may die on the lips that gave it—yet some soul, somewhere, shall catch the refrain and echo it down the ages.

The success of this book will be proportional to the numbers that do not read it—now. And its failure may be measured by the amount of applause it calls forth. Give me a hearing—but spare me an audience. Open your ears and your hearts to me— but close your eyes and your lips. Take what little good there may be here for you, and leave the rest. Do not question me. Do not praise me. Above all, do not detain me. This is but a glimpse of Truth. And I cannot pause while still the horizon widens and the sun gains in glory.

A PERSONAL PROLOGUE

Words in themselves are as futile as stray bricks.

They endure only when cemented by feeling and aligned by purpose. The field of literature is mostly a dreary brick-yard, with chipped and broken bits scattered about to mark what might have been had the builder known.

Life is the only literature that lives. And if I had not first lived this book, it would never be worth the writing. *To write for any other reason than that one must* is to insult oneself and to martyr one's friends. If you write only when you must, you may not always be considerate to your friends. But you will at least be true to yourself. And the perusal of your writings can never be too hard a price to pay for knowing some one who is sincere. Sincere humans are about as common as brave gazelles or compassionate tigers.

"The Philosophy of Fasting" is a plea for human sincerity and a treatise on human wholeness. The first twenty-five years of my life I was anything but whole. Because I was anything but sincere. I did not dare be true to myself, or with my fellows. Civilization, classicism and orthodoxy had combined to make me appear what I was not and crucify what I was. Body, brain and soul, I was burdened with a mass of externals that weighed heavier and sunk deeper day by day, until the life was almost crushed out of me.

Born a weakling, I was a semi-invalid and chronic sufferer during most of my boyhood and youth. Some fifteen forms of constitutional disease took turns troubling me; until family, friends and physicians began to despair of the outcome. At one time I was taking six kinds of medicine, weighed 110 pounds instead of 150, spent most of the time beside the fire, or on the couch, and threatened to become useless to myself and everybody else. The ailments were chiefly nervous and digestive, and were caused by inequalities of make-up. Inheriting from my father a brain incessantly active, from my mother a soul supersensitive and a physique small and tremulous, from both an insatiable ambition; I seemed unable to balance myself at all. Wearing a man's hat at twelve, I had the body of a boy of eight, with a soul older than any I had ever met. Naturally no one understood me. And the greatest puzzle to me in the Universe was I to myself.

I could not ride in a carriage, sit in a hammock, or climb a tree without growing dizzy, sick and faint. The slightest physical jar or mental irritation brought on headaches that lasted for days. Public gatherings oppressed and stifled me—it was the poisonous insincerity of social usage, though I did not know it then.

The routine of existence was eternally maddening me— every clock, calendar and school-bell in town seemed to shriek the cruelty of law and order. The claim of senseless customs, the grasp of useless habits, the sway of rule and rote, the clutter of superfluous possessions, the onus of fictitious duties, the miasma of popular opinion, the rut of precedent, the chain of environment, the blindfold of superstition;—from all these barriers to human progress I was struggling to be free. The doctors meanwhile declared with oracular accent they could find no physiological basis for disease—it must be all in my imagination!

Of course it was. Everything is that counts. And especially a doctor's diagnosis—which counts financially.

Let us abridge this recital of symptoms, and pass on to the cure.

As a last recourse, I tried Physical Culture. Studied and applied to myself various systems of Dietetics, Hydrotherapy, Dynamic Breathing, Movement Methods Active and Passive, Sun, Air and Earth Cure, and other modes of Naturopathy.

These all helped. Fully half of my ailments presently disappeared. But the mind and soul were not so easily satisfied. So I took up Suggestion, Mental Science, New Thought, Oriental

Philosophy, and kindred quasi-religious faiths. But they were all more or less man-made. And I had to have God.

Then came the Thirty-Day Fast. I found God through this Fast. Which is equivalent to saying I found Myself. For We are One and the Same. During this month I ate nothing at all, drank nothing but water and occasionally acid fruit-juice. There were four objects to be achieved by means of this rather heroic measure:—*Renovation, Delectation, Domination, Illumination.* Every one was realized. Physically, I was healthier than for ten years before. Sensuously, I enjoyed everything as I had done when a child. Mentally, I got a grip on myself that nothing had ever given and that nothing now can ever shake. Spiritually, I saw the heavens opened and the ultimate truths of the Infinite revealed in glorious array beyond the span of the sunrise or the gleam of the farthest star.

You can do the same. Or more. All you need is supreme faith in yourself, exact knowledge of the method, and steadfast purpose, to realize the highest prophecy stored for you in the archives of the Almighty. I will give you the knowledge, Omnipotence will give you the faith, so all you must supply is the purpose. Which comes of itself—with a vision of the possibilities.

Fasting is not a panacea.

Only Nature grants panaceas. And she makes hers fresh for each case. Nor does she employ human dispensaries.

But Fasting, *rightly conducted and completed,* is nearest a panacea for all mortal ills of any drugless remedy I know, whether physiological, metaphysical, or inspirational. Fasting, resting, airing, bathing, breathing, exercising and hoping—these seven simple measures, if *sanely* proportioned and administered, will cure any case of acute disease. And almost any case of chronic.

It is not however with the therapeutic side we are chiefly concerned in this book. The healing phase is unquestionably the most vital. But its importance has caused it to be discussed already in a variety of convincing ways by specialist pioneers, preceding me in the field. *"The Philosophy of Fasting"* considers rather the mental, psychic and spiritual components which are themselves based on the physiological.

This work therefore should be deemed supplementary to the following five books in particular:

1. "The No-Breakfast Plan and Fasting Cure." By Dr. Edward Hooker Dewey. Published by Author at Meadville, Pennsylvania.
2. "Fasting, Hydropathy and Exercise." By Dr. Felix Oswald and Bernarr Macfadden. Published by Physical Culture Publishing Co.—Spotswood, New Jersey.
3. "The A. B.-Z. of Our Own Nutrition." By Horace Fletcher. Published by Frederic A. Stokes Co.—New York City.
4. "Perfect Health." By C. C. Haskell. Published by Author at Norwich, Connecticut.
5. "Return to Nature." By Adolf Just. Published by Naturopathic Publishing Co.—124 East 59th Street, New York City.

There are several reasons why these other authors should be read first. In this book of mine I have given almost no biological facts, experimental data, or scientific proofs. I appeal to the heart, the soul, and the consciousness more than to the brain.

It is a pathetic truism however that the only part of most people anywhere near alive is this same brain I would subordinate. Their axiomatic perceptions are hopelessly dulled. And they can't be convinced of the most overwhelming truth save by some such roundabout route as an affidavit or syllogism.

Now these treatises aforementioned abound in substantial facts—facts physical, logical and historical. Doctor Dewey and Mr. Fletcher in particular have devoted much time, thought, energy, altruism and persistence to *demonstrating* their own beautiful theories of life, health and happiness.

I have proved to myself everything I put in print. But I'm not desirous of converting anybody else. And I haven't time to retrace the line of travel in order to describe it. So, to satisfy your brain as well as your soul—and it's just as necessary—you will be wise to take first the facts offered you by more patient investigators.

Another thing. Progress is best when it's gradual. You don't knock out all the underpinning of a house you're moving —you gently abstract one prop after another. One drawback to this book is it doesn't leave you any props at all—props medicinal, metaphysical, social, conventional, moral, theological, or otherwise respectable. And it'll be easier for you to feel them fall by degrees, with a nicety more mercifully adjusted.

One more statement, and then this very tedious prologue is at an end. It's about the little essays which comprise the greater part of the book. They have two reasons for being.

In the first place, this matter of Fasting bears directly on every one of the thirteen themes presented. It doesn't take long to show the connection. But to define the author's understanding of terms is a lengthier and more difficult problem. Because it is not the common conception at all, in the majority of cases.

Secondly, the man who publishes this book is the only one I have yet found with sufficient courage to print the things I believe. We don't think altogether alike. And he isn't responsible for anything I say. But we both esteem sincerity first of all, come what may as a consequence. Mr. Lust, moreover, as sponsor of the *Naturopathic Idea,* offers the broadest basis yet presented for the upbuilding of Human Wholeness.

This therefore seems a good opportunity to express certain beliefs that demand to be expressed for the sake of the expressing.

In conclusion, I commend to you very earnestly not the author—not the theory—not the book; solely, utterly and everlastingly, Truth. Only when Truth and a mortal coincide, does the mortal become immortal. I would not have it otherwise if I could. And my one hope is that enough of the splendor of immortality may shine through this message to light you a little farther up the steeps of attainment.

Edward Earle Purinton.

New York City, December first, nineteen hundred and five.

FASTING FOR HEALTH

CHAPTER I.

"To be healthy is to be half-animal and half-god; to be sickly is to be circumscribedly human; but to be sane is to be triunely god-man-animal."

In clarification whereof is this book written.

A whole book to explain a whole sentence? And why not? Libraries have been evolved upon a foundation of three short words, namely "Life is protoplasm." Yet who can define Life, or analyze protoplasm?

In this opening sentence of mine there is blended all the subtlety of metaphysics with all the simplicity of childhood. By a little effort you may perhaps penetrate the realm of Mind; but ah! who, tell me who, can fathom a child?

The last place to look for sanity is in a sanitarium; the next to the last in a health resort.

To be sanitary is not necessarily to be *sane—Saneness* being the one word that sums this book. If we had always lived sanely, we should never need sanitation. In the Reformers' Stiff-legged Race for Popularity, hygienic hobbies are at present in the lead. Their name is legion, and each ridden more recklessly than all the rest. You'd think surely they must collide —until you remember that *hobbies never advance.* In this respect are hygienic hobbies as docile as their lay brethren who haven't any "mission" but just to be wood painted red.

Far be it from me to ridicule any man who believes he has a mission. Such are the world's saviors. I myself have a mission—a part of it being to deliver the world from health cranks. I was a health crank once. Some of you may doubt the past tense — but you should have seen me then! I am haunted yet by the look of dread on the faces of my friends as they saw me approaching from afar. Whereas now, you can at least interpolate a wan smile occasionally.

I assume at the outset that you have read the books suggested in the Prologue; that you are more or less at home in various branches of Naturism—Dietetics, Hydrotherapy, Lung and Muscle Culture, Suggestion, and the like; that, having read the Prologue, you are prepared to be patient with the author; and that, having learned through suffering to be sincere, you will be able to recognize sincerity of motive—however faulty be the method.

First a few incoherent remarks on Health in general.

Pill-time is only pallor-time. And the puzzle is to remove the pallor, yet leave the pill in the box. The druggist never solves it—he makes the patient swallow the pill. The Naturist almost never solves it—he summarily smashes the pill-box but forgets to look at the face of the patient. I did that once— threw the patient's pill-box out of the car-window. He was kind of new to Naturism, just coming to take treatment. When he saw all his concentrated hopes of health vanished forever, he rushed to a telegraph office before I could stop him; wired a friend three hundred miles off to come quick—he was dying; then collapsed into a comatosé of despair. He didn't die. He got completely well, went home and cured his whole family connection of whatever ailed them. He cured *me* of something, too—of throwing away a patient's pill-box. That's a lesson every Naturist must learn in order to succeed. Most of them haven't learned it—and most of them don't succeed. Understand, drugs can't cure. Drugs kill—always. *But.*

Drugs are useful so long as they *help a man's mind more* than they *harm* his *body*. This the best physicians recognize, being Naturists in belief—but wise enough to keep still about it. If the patient believes in drugs and his doctor doesn't, the patient lives; if the patient doesn't and his doctor does, the patient dies. The virtue of any medicine being directly proportional to its faith and inversely proportional to its substance.

Here again is the eternal paradox of Truth verified, since

drug-cure is faith-cure. People *believe* they must "take something" so long as they *believe* they can "catch something." Nature-cure requires no faith—only sincerity; a Kneipp douche or Kuhne sitzbath will clear out disease whether the sick man believes or not.

A momentary digression.

You may have observed I begin certain impersonal words with capitals. I always begin Nature, Truth and Love with large letters. Because Nature is my mother, Truth is my teacher, and Love is my God.

Disease is a godsend. Never to be dreaded, always to be esteemed beneficent. How microbes are maligned, to be sure. A microbe is a sort of somatic undertaker, his business being to dispose of the dead among the cells. The trouble is we all array ourselves in black and join the mourners at the funeral. Away with funerals! Away with mourning! Away with the *earthiness* of superstition! For superstition is always earthy, instead of religious as men suppose.

The danger in all disease lies in the remedy, and not in the ailment. Left alone, disease would cure itself, through the instinct of the invalid. But the human race is a race of meddlers. Certain highly-respected classes have actually reduced meddling to a science, and make their living by it. Such as lawyers, who interfere between man and man; doctors, who interfere between man and Nature; and preachers, who interfere between man and God. So we have our "bitter medicine"—of therapeutics and theology, the claim being that the worse a thing tastes the better it is, and we should swallow it for no other conceivable reason but that we don't want to. We have also our School of Hysterical Hygiene, most health reformers serving ex-officio on the Faculty. These begoggled brethren tell us many curious and marvelous tales, tales imported from Liliput and Brobdingnag.

They tell us for instance to drink just two glasses of water on arising, exactly one-and-a-half on retiring, and one, to the drop, every hour between. A harmless occupation that—for a man who has nothing better to do than wander anxiously about all day with a clock in one hand and a water-cooler in the other.

They tell us *never* to drink when eating. Nature doesn't tell us that. Nature says, "Drink only and always when thirsty."

They tell us to chew each mouthful thirty, forty or fifty times by the metronome; and not dare swallow a morsel till we've looked up in the book whether it will agree with every morsel gone before. Gracious me, if we have to write the biography of each bite as it passes, when do we get time to enjoy our food? Mince-pie served with a smile is quite as hygienic as raw wheat served with a scowl.

They tell us to take the Milk-Cure, if we would level our corporeal ravines. Well, a porker is fat. And I suppose that by similar process, a man might be fattened—though I should hate to think it of a woman. You know what *pâté de foies gras* is made of, don't you? If you fancy that sort of provender, you better take the Milk-and-Egg-Cure to the limit.

They tell us to repeat certain prescribed "Affirmations" three times a day and on going to bed. With a metaphysical emergency case handy, put up by somebody of the name of Wilmans, or Towne, or Eddy, or Atkinson. Well, a *bread* pill is easier to remember.

They tell us to measure so many inches crosswise for a corresponding number up-and-down-wise; and to tip the beam precisely on the dot of a specified ounce. So? Yes, yes, a woman *may* be a wax figure, a man *may* be an anatomical model. But not all, not all. A few of us are individuals. And for such there are no standards, anthropomorphic or otherwise. No standards dietetic, gymnastic, metaphysical, social, political, ethical, or religious. Nothing anywhere but the soul and the Infinite—and the means on earth to blend the two.

I don't like satire or sarcasm.

My heart tells me my brain hasn't any business to go bumping into people like that. But still, when they get in the way and you're in a hurry, what are you to do? I guess I'm a good deal like the impetuous mother that castigates her child and then gives it sugar-plums to stop its crying. Because I want to say that all these vagaries of Naturism or New Thought contain more Truth than error; while the leaders who propagate reform theories are without exception benefactors to the race. Their eyes may be skewed; but their hearts are right and their work is redemption. Which same could perhaps be said of me—I don't know.

Now for the Fast.

An extreme Fast—say from twenty to forty days, is just as apt to wreck a man as it is to rescue him. Unless, as I have mentioned before, it be *properly conducted and completed.* In this book I can but touch on the physiological side. That however has been amply and accurately covered by Doctor Dewey, Mr. Macfadden, Mr. Fletcher, and Mr. Haskell. Better than I could do it — far better. And yet their very thoroughness *as scientists* has incapacitated them for keen soul-perception. So that they have mostly overlooked the mental, psychic and spiritual phases. Which in the long view are vastly more important than the physical.

Sane Fasting never injured anybody—*sanitary* Fasting has often done it. And people shrink from the Fast because of the follies that usually accompany it. Milton Rathbun for instance —Doctor Dewey's star case—fasted thirty-five days, then made his first meal of *oysters, soda crackers, beef broth and Oolong tea.* All of which iniquities a *really hungry man cannot crave.* If the pupil of so famous a teacher didn't clarify his instinct any better than that, what could you expect from common folks, uninstructed and uninspired?

Fasting in itself is purely a negative process.

It must be *supplemented* by a *positive regime.*

There are only two excuses for taking a crutch from a cripple; when you can give him a better, or when he can stand alone. The whole human race is crippled. And their crutch is the food-habit. Be careful, brother, how you attempt to remove it. Have you a substitute men can *use?*

I know people who have acquired the Fast-habit. They starve about a third of the time. Just as foolish as to eat all the time. And a lot more uncomfortable.

Having once solved the Personal Equation in Wholeness, you need not resort to the Fast, unless you care to. But how many have solved it? Perhaps a score of humans—since time began. The greatest Messiah that has thus far voiced his message *had* to take the extreme Fast, to get perfectly clear. And I have yet to find the Freethinker who is more worthy of emulation than Jesus, the Master Christ. Not of imitation, mind. If all of God outside of me were to incarnate suddenly into one colossal Being and appear thus stupendous in Its might, think you I should bow the knee? The God in my own soul would rise majestic and answer calmly, "I am Your Equal."

Fasting is not merely denying oneself food—I don't believe in self-denial. Self is God. Self-denial is therefore blasphemy. The extreme Fast must be based upon, and adapted to, *some dominant purpose.* Most people fast with the sole idea of cleansing their bodies. I call that starving—not Fasting. And to distinguish what I consider the real Fast, that taken *sanely* and with a *four-fold motive,* I have given it throughout this book a special name. I call it

"THE CONQUEST FAST."

Whenever therefore you find this term, you will recognize the Fast designated by this book and no other.

The first surprising statement to be made of the Conquest Fast for health of body is this: *I do not recommend it.*

It ensures health of body quicker than any other one measure of Naturism. But *not to those who put health of body above health of mind and soul.* For purely therapeutic purposes, a number of short Fasts would be better, ranging from two to seven days each, and occurring at intervals of say three times their own duration. Moreover their effect will usually be enhanced if you take acid fruit-juice unsweetened, in addition to pure water. The juice of a half-dozen oranges a day, or three lemons diluted, or half a pint of grape-juice in a pint of water; such gentle febrifuge, stimulant, laxative and germicide will hasten physical recovery perceptibly. Indeed a strict fresh fruit dietary adhered to for a week or two every Spring and Fall would almost obviate any need for a Fast at any time.

Assuming however that we believe in the unity indivisible of body, mind and soul, nor would attempt to perfect one at the expense of the others, let us ask wherein the Conquest Fast directly heightens health of body.

From experience I cull a few out of the many benefits you also would realize.

1. *The Conquest Fast solves finally and forever that most perplexing problem — "What shall I eat?"* This is the first question a sick man asks—and the last one a well man answers. You ask it for yourself, you must answer it from yourself. Answers from without only bewilder you. The wisest dietist on earth—and there isn't any yet—could do no more than give you data you must *forget* before you eat sanely. I have studied, practiced—and *disproved for me,* a score of the most popular dietetic theories. So long as they keep to physiological *fact* they are useful. But the moment they add *inference and generalization* —that moment they verge on fallacy. Most men, for instance, are undoubtedly herbivorous by nature. They are sheep—they should eat grass. Still I know men who are lions. Such demand meat. Whether a lion or a lamb be further up in the scale of evolution we will leave to the verdict in that famous case, *New York Vegetarian Society* vs. *New York Evening Journal.* Each of these disputants is final authority—and each calls the other imbecile.

Back to the Fast—back quick; I guess I must have been cut out for a preacher after all. First though let us bid fond farewell to the gastronomic proselyters. In a chunk of advice on how to give advice under all circumstances;—"Go into another room and whisper it."

Hearken ye to the Conquest Fast.

Eat always and only what Instinct tells you; but be sure it IS Instinct speaking.

Let me illustrate. When I was in College, I ate mostly mush. This was perhaps excusable since all the facts they made me swallow were dry as dust. But it wasn't wholesome, it wasn't natural. I liked gravies, sauces, custards and puddings with an unholy liking. I used to sneak off on my bicycle to the nearest bake-shop, seven miles distant, where fat cream-puffs were to be had cheap. Salving my conscience by saving one—the smallest and emptiest—for my little sister. I didn't care for fruits and vegetables—but I reveled in fried liver and hot soda biscuits. Particularly was salt essential to me—I would entomb it till the tears came.

Note the revolution wrought by the Fast. I *wasn't hungry at all through the first three weeks*—whereas before I never could get enough; overeating is the commonest cause of starvation, let us remark in passing. When I began to gravitate slowly toward the cupboard, along about the twenty-fifth day, I found two-thirds of the foods there were actually impossible for me to eat. Yet *all* were hygienic, well-prepared, pure. They simply wouldn't satisfy *my individual hunger*—a hunger I hadn't known before, since babyhood. Nuts and fruits I craved most, with a few vegetables and natural grains a close second. *Nothing else.* Fried foods nauseated me. Ice-cream soda was so much swill. "Dainties" usually thrust on an invalid seemed but sickening imitations of nutriment. The very thought of "cream-puffs"— and I did recall the soggy things—made me shudder. Salt was as superfluous as star-dust; I don't care for it now even on eggs. Instinct was once more alive and active. In point of hunger at least I was a perfect animal—first. Note this also; I didn't want any Grape-Nuts, Malted Milk, or Protose Steak, such concoctions being sanitary but not sane. Since the Fast, I have never hesitated for one moment over what to eat. *I always know.* Do you?

2. *The Conquest Fast simplifies diagnosis.* Do you really

know what ails you?   Does the doctor?   Does anybody?   I always know what ails me—if anything does; and *exactly how* to remedy it.   A few months ago I had the measles.   A severe case, too.   Resulting from the unnaturalness of city life, which I am at present undergoing for a purpose.   I was absolutely alone during the whole ten days of illness, save for a few hours when a friend happened in.   I not only knew what to do for myself—I did it. And delirious half the time, at that. A doctor's diagnosis? What for?

A doctor's diagnosis is the first rehearsal for that tragedy known as the Post-mortem Examination.   If he doesn't say it right (and a doctor stammers by profession), he calls in a surgeon to prompt him;—together they enact the final rehearsal with an operating-table for a stage.   Then all they need for a perfect performance is the corpse.   Which usually arrives in good time.

During a long Fast, you learn for yourself what's the matter with you.   Both physically and psychically.   Because the Fast reaches direct the three vital centres whence all disturbance arises —Digestion, Thought and Sex.   The Conquest Fast *rejuvenates,* whereas common measures of Naturopathy only *renovate.*

3. *The Conquest Fast conserves vital force.*   Other systems tend to waste it.   Gymnastics for instance, or the Water-Cure.   "Healed while you wait"—that's Fasting.   More—healed while you rest; healed while you regain the instincts, desires and sensibilities of childhood.   A point not to be overlooked by the American, so proverbially spendthrift of his energies.   Just be still and trust Nature.

4. *The Conquest Fast dispels therapeutic errors,* saving thereby valuable time, thought, and financial outlay.   Three examples.   (*a*). *There is no such thing as "brain food"*—either fish or phosphates.   The less food, the clearer brain; the purer food, the stronger brain; that's all. (*b*). *Nothing can cure disease that does not also enhance health.*   Medicine does neither—the Conquest Fast does both.   In short, "Specifics" are absurd; whether for brain alone, soul alone, or body alone in whole or

in part. (*c*). *You needn't "travel for your health"*—that's the wrong direction, health residing equally beneath you and above you. Where Nature is, there is health. Where civilization is, there is disease. Be less human, more natural, more divine; this is the clue to saneness. Take your mind off your symptoms and put it on your soul. Break through human barriers. Transcend human limitations. Learn of the animals—and *live* as the animals do. Learn of the gods—and *love* as the gods do. Learn of the human immortals who have dared do both these things, facing simultaneously the world's present condemnation, with its eternal gratitude echoing through the future.

"To be healthy is to be half-animal and half-god; to be sickly is to be circumscribedly human; but to be *sane* is to be triunely god-man-animal."

Naturism may make you half-animal.

Divine Science may make you half-god.

Nothing can make you so completely *yourself,* god-man-animal you were born to be, as the Conquest Fast with what should ensue therefrom.

Don't believe my word.

Don't believe anything you haven't lived and proved. But *be willing to believe*—for your own sake, not for mine.

Man's *one irredeemable errcr* is to scoff at what he cannot understand and will not investigate.

FASTING FOR ENJOYMENT

CHAPTER II.

Warning to deep thinkers: *your risibles need exercising as much as your plausibles.* Besides, you'd look more attractive.

This applies to health cranks also. .Whenever you see the face of a health crank fall, by all means let it drop! Heaven knows he needs a new one.

You say there's nothing to smile at? Oh, yes, there is. Listen. How to have a constant source of amusement; *learn to laugh at yourself.* Every human deserves to be laughed at about so much—if you do it for yourself, you relieve your neighbor of the necessity. And it's more comfortable for you.

People won't follow a long face—a full moon looks more inviting than a hatchet. *Reform fails because it frowns.* It worships Duty instead of Desire. You have a perfect right to say, "Damn Duty!" Because to damn Duty is to deify Desire— at least it should be.

My duty is what the other fellow thinks I should do because he wouldn't if he were I. I'd be a chump to do it. I don't like that word "chump;" it doesn't sound nice. But while we're talking of disagreeable things, we might as well bunch them.

Back to Reform for a minute. Not more than a minute— the atmosphere is too malarial. Tammany wins and the Anti-Vice Society loses. Why? Truth never loses. Love never loses. God never loses. I'll tell you why. Because the presbyopic Parkhurstians have forgotten this cardinal principle: that *whatever is natural is also delightful.* They are a vestige of the austerities of the Dark Ages—something like the dodo or ichthyosaurus; if only they were as fast approaching extinction!

Reform calls the people together with the exhorter's fire-bell of eternal torment; then struts vaingloriously in their front for two hours, proclaiming raucously that dismal doctrine of "Thou Shalt Not." Meanwhile Tammany has sought out the tenements that house but do not shelter the poor; has rapped softly on the door; has asked gently "How's your coal-bin to-day?

Has the doctor been paid? We're to have a little celebration to-morrow, with popcorn and candy for the children; you will come, won't you?"

Wise Tammany. Stupid Reform.

Would you reach a man's soul? Feed his stomach, clothe his back, and warm his heart. Don't bother his brain—nothing is so dangerous for most men as to begin to think. Body and heart are one with soul, whereas brain is mostly an interloper. *Tammany alternates the wisdom of God with the follies of Man —the Anti-Vicers manifest neither.* Scant choice indeed. But what little there is goes to Tammany. Any Naturist will tell you eczema is easier to cure than anaemia.

The reason the world won't be reformed is because it shouldn't be. It should be instructed—and inspired. But most of all *smiled upon.* The world wants Truth. The world does not want the *errors, deficiencies and excesses of the professional exponents of Truth.* Whenever you find a man complaining that people won't accept his message, you find a man whose message is incomplete.

Do you like hurdy-gurdies?

I do—they call the little children to dance on the sidewalk. I'd join them myself; only the stiff, sallow, wizened grown-ups preserving their dignity in the carbonic acid gas of a hermetically sealed house would think I was crazy and hurry the children in. Carbonic acid gas is a good preservative for dignity. When dignity has become fixed, we call it death.

My, what a jump—from reform to hurdy-gurdy. Doesn't it feel fine to be out in the sunlight again? The play-spirit is irrepressible in the young of all animals. Watch a kitten, a lamb, a little squirrel, a healthy baby. Then observe an aggregation of the elite, sorted, starched and polished for a society function. No wonder they need monkeys for guests of honor—we always honor those wiser than ourselves.

I remember how it was when I was a boy—it's all right to get over being a *boy,* provided you remain a *child.* I couldn't dig potatoes in the hot sun ten minutes without getting a raging headache. But I could outstay a four-hour stretch of tennis that same day, and still be chipper at the close. My family misjudged me—they called me "constitutionally tired." I wasn't lazy—I was only natural. Potatoes aren't natural; you don't have to dig berries off bushes or nuts off trees. Things God plants grow skyward. (Suppose a small boy should see this, about ten o'clock in the morning, with company coming for dinner, and no potatoes dug! But you can't get at me, you poor flurried mother—because you haven't my address. Still I'm a little scared—I was once in the boy's trousers. What a wonderful thing memory is! [Or maybe it's only imagination. Because you mustn't infer that the parental discipline of manual juxta-position prevailed in our family. My parents were always most lenient with my abnormalities and tolerant of my digressions.])

Speaking of youth, I know some people who hope to live exactly one hundred years. They have formed a Club for that purpose. I went to one of their meetings. I didn't go again—I don't like funerals. They were merely holding a wake over their own defunct hearts. What's the use? Spectres aren't supposed to die anyway. A tortoise lives a hundred years; who wants a tortoise for a bed-fellow?

We haven't lost sight of the Conquest Fast—we're just viewing the surrounding scenery.

You read in the annals of the church how many weeks a certain saint fasted. And you image to yourself a lugubrious visage, with cadaverous cheeks, compressed lips, aquiline features, furrowed brow, haunted eyes, pallid flesh; and the whole grim calamity surmounted by a thick black cowl.

Now that isn't my picture at all.

I smile more than I frown. No cowl ever made could abash my hair—it's a cross between Elbert Hubbard's and Paderewski's. And my lips are the kind to kiss with. Baby-kisses, you stupid man. If you always had baby-kisses in your mouth, your sweetheart would have some other kind in hers. But since you don't know anything about baby-kisses, and they are the most needed, she has to supply them all.

I don't like these personalities any more than you do. But they prove I am human. Whereas most of the souls that have distanced Humanity have also forgotten the way back.

Asceticism and sensualism are equally unnatural. The ascetic would refine his body. He is right. The sensualist would enjoy his body. Also right. But each makes the mistake of being anti-the-other. Don't be *anti*-anything, be simply *non*. Sooner or later every knocker pounds his own thumb.

Pain is the penalty for forcing pleasure; death is the penalty for denying it. To enjoy life is to use naturally every natural function of life; not to think too much or to feel too little. Happiness is the unsought crown bestowed on self-fidelity. And it rests so light we never know it's there.

To eat *for* pleasure is to eat for pain; but to eat *without* pleasure is to eat without life. Soul suffers most when body seeks enjoyment for itself. Indeed *the only sense-pleasures that cause regret are those which the soul failed to feel first.* In short, soul-hunger can never be surfeited; and *all hunger should be soul-hunger.*

Here is a sure remedy for indigestion: eat a very little of whatever you love best, and enjoy it to the utmost. No one ever loved too much; even excess of passion is lack of Love.

Work for the joy of working, play for the joy of playing, eat for the joy of eating—and *fast for the joy of fasting.*

I have been asked "How, in the name of all that is mystical, can you *fast* for enjoyment?" Well, a materialist can't. But a materialist won't ever undertake a Conquest Fast. So such are eliminated. Only he will enjoy the Fast who *can* enjoy *both soul and sense.*

Let me give you the secret of enjoyment in six words: *minimum of real, maximum of ideal.* Nothing that we have sublimized can satiate us. It satisfies—but stops there. Let Deity invest the mortal, and the mortal blossoms into immortality.

To sense the sweetness of a flower, look within its heart—not upon the dumb clay that clots its external.

If you fail to enjoy life, it is because you are living on the surface. And even the Almighty is often incompetent to smoothe the surface of things. Your blood is sluggish, your organs are clogged, your nerves are deadened, your brain is confused, your heart is chilled, your senses are numb; your soul is stifling.

During the Conquest Fast, you should be happier everywhere save in two small patches of your anatomy—your palate and your brain. But they don't deserve to be happy—they have been insubordinate too long. After the first week or so, discomfort vanishes here also.

It might be well to state that during the first week of the Fast, the enjoyment of your friends and neighbors will not be particularly enhanced. They'll make it worse for you and you for them. By referring to the Twenty Rules however, you will see a way around this omen.

We are told by our friends the metaphysicians that Happiness is Harmony. If that be so, you will find yourself growing supremely happy toward the close of a two-weeks', three-weeks', or four-weeks' Fast. Every fibre of your body will be attuned to Nature, every quiver of your soul made seraphic with its melody of Truth. That long-lost child-sensibility will steal over you once more, a child being proverbially happy *because its soul is fed on the finer forces* of earth and air and ether; forces cut off from men by their grosser environs of civilization.

Is this kind of enjoyment too mystical?

All right, we'll have some that isn't. You should have seen me eat at the close of my Thirty-Day Fast! Delight— rapture — ecstacy — transport — bliss — all beggarly words to describe the sensation.

Just between me and you—I'll have to whisper it, for I wouldn't have anybody else hear for the world;—but if I were a rank materialist, caring nothing about soul, I should fast awhile just for the fun of eating when hungry. I recall how a College Professor used to do that—he taught in the University that made a lumber-room out of me. He was a "D.D." too—D.D. standing for "Death's Deputy." Thanksgiving morning he used to stay home from church so as to play tennis and get a whaling appetite for Turkey. He had boils to pay for it, so he did. I'm not blaming this particular Professor—indeed he was broader and saner than the majority. It's something for a classicist to appreciate the value of an appetite—if he did go at it wrong.

Fasting—*then Feasting.*

That's my doctrine.

Cream once a week instead of milk-and-water every day. Some folks can't digest cream. But I have a shy suspicion it's because they won't fast. They'd rather be half-way comfortable in their bodies than altogether sane in their souls. Of course they're anaemic—even a baby sickens on watered milk. Don't try to wean them. When they're grown enough, Nature will send them foraging for themselves.

Happiness is like a rare species of butterfly—seldom caught and sure to die in captivity. But if you are very, very still, it may alight near you; where you can revel in the golden lustre of its wings, the subtle poise of its body, the matchless grace of its flight.

And then good-bye. Good-bye.

FASTING FOR FREEDOM

CHAPTER III.

Habit is the "Family-Entrance" to that notorious resort called Hell.

Most of the people who go there use this side-door.

For two reasons. First, because it is supposed to be more respectable than that broad, front, pendulum-portal of *Abandon.* Second, because the policeman is always looking the other way. His name is Law, and he is paid to watch just the front entrance. I have this only by hearsay, not being acquainted with him personally. You see when Love and I go trysting together we always take the opposite direction—the road that leads to Heaven. Love says she can't bear the sight of Law—he makes her tremble all over. So I have come to avoid him myself. Since Love's feminine intuition is the nearest infallible of anything in this world.

I do not exaggerate in thus defining Habit.

Analyze all the crime, disease, and misfortune among men, and you trace it to a habit. Drink-habit, drug-habit, food-habit, passion-habit, worry-habit, gossip-habit, fear-habit, greed-habit, credulity-habit, hypocrisy-habit,—and health-food-habit; these with a hundred more of their close kin are directly to blame for Humanity's blind bondage to the surface form of things.

The human body should be bound by no habits save those decreed by animal instinct. The human mind should be bound by no habits save those required in its quest for Truth. The human soul should be bound by no habits save those that iterate its own inspiration. To think for oneself, to act for oneself, most of all to *feel* for oneself; this is to outgrow, overtop, and bury in oblivion the habits of the race.

The only harmless habit is that newly-created by a self-conscious soul for its own individual use. No other habit is based on absolute sincerity. I was once a Republican—because my father was; a Baptist—because my mother was; a classicist—because my teacher was; a beefsteak-eater—because my cook was; and a Sunday-School scholar—because John D. Rockefeller, Junior, posed as official class-exhorter. Needless to say I was "doped" all through—pardon the slang.

I am now a Cosmocrat. Which is a new word. There was none big enough before. It both includes and excludes the petty minor distinctions of party, class and creed that once made of a cosmic mind a mere collection of cubby-holes.

Even the freedom-habit becomes bad when you can't break it. You may get your message on the mountain-peak, but only in the valley can you give it. Since deaf is the world to voices from on high, blind is the world to visions celestial.

Man, the only being with the upturned face, is the only being with the downcast eye. Is it not pitiful?

My conscience is pricking me. I'll have to confess to *one* bad habit. The note-book habit. I've jotted down enough memoranda to make a library. That's where most of the epigrams in this book come from. After all, I'm not the one to suffer on account of this habit, am I? Only my readers.

I started to compile a Catalogue of Bad Human Habits; with Cures and Preventives therefor.

But the job soon grew to be hopeless. So we'll just cite a few, taken from the list at random. Everybody does these things because everybody else does. Whereas nobody wants to, nobody should. Generally speaking.

BAD HUMAN HABITS

(To be found in your next-door neighbor)

Arguing	Imitating	Posing	Doubting
Interfering	Begging	Boasting	Punishing
Advising	Borrowing	Pretending	Avenging
Complaining	Wishing	Hesitating	Proselyting
Nagging	Boosting	Hurrying	Economizing
Tagging	Defending	Agitating	Mourning
Lopping	Explaining	Reforming	Dreading
Propping	Straddling	Exhorting	Condoling

Misconstruing motives
Over-eating (chief of them all)
Over-fasting (not epidemic)
"Catching" diseases
"Taking something" for them
Running for the doctor (instead of from)
Discussing food
Sitting around for meal-time
Urging our friends to eat
"Cultivating an appetite"
Trying to eat, drink, talk and truckle simultaneously
Wearing flannels
Airing our ailments
Consorting with health hobbyists
Watching the clock
"Holding down" a job
Running the government
"Paying" social calls
Reading newspapers
Going to church
Attending funerals and weddings
Naming the baby
Wilting at the weather
Wearing custom-made clothes and opinions
Persisting in **regular** correspondence
Slandering rivals
Owning friends
Heaping abuse on the rich
Heaping charity on the poor
Deploring mistakes
Vaunting victories
Counting our "mercies"
Sandpapering our injuries
Idolizing the brain
Ridiculing what we don't understand
Teaching literature rather than Life
Imputing wisdom to doctors, preachers and professors
Belittling manual work

Bowing to authority
Pandering to public opinion
Letting "honor" outrank honesty
Wearing a label
Eulogizing consistency
Pitying anybody — ourselves in particular
Persecuting pioneers
Despising dreamers
Frowning on enthusiasm
Cherishing outgrown ideals
Judging Genius
Sullying Sex
Denying Desire
Obeying Duty
Decreeing marriage moral
Dictating to the individual
Maligning the "lower animals"
Condemning sin
Being painfully good
Pressing tracts and plug hats on the "heathen"
Strewing a grave with flowers
Surfeiting warriors—and starving poets
Jumping at conclusions
Forgetting how to laugh
Esteeming speech more than silence
Taking pride in personality
Fearing to act on impulse
Exalting reason above instinct
Threatening and scolding children
Remaining strangers to the hills, the sea, and the stars
Worshipping man, god or devil
Imagining Truth can lead astray
Preferring dishonest orthodoxy to honest heresy
Divorcing God and Nature
Relying on faith alone, or fact alone
Prizing form more than Spirit
Forcing or crushing Love
Silencing the voice of the Soul

Did you survive?

Then, after a little breathing-spell, we'll continue.

While you're resting, you might send to the Naturopathic Publishing Company, 124 East Fifty-ninth Street, New York City, for back numbers of *"The Naturopath"*, *December,* 1902 *to March,* 1903 inclusive. Enclosing say twenty cents. These issues of this Magazine contain articles written by me on "The Folly of the Food-Habit," suggesting therefrom the wisdom of the Fast. I don't entirely agree with the sentiments of so long ago—when my pen was wont to picture everything jet black with a lurid lining. But if you will refer to them, it will save a duplicate recital here of pessimistic anarchism. Iconoclasm may demolish the ruins of error—only Idealism can build the structure of Truth. Be very sure every iconoclast sees more error than Truth.

Small men are "creatures of habit"—great men are creators of habit. This explains hero-worship. Since creature always worships creator. Either we make our habits or our habits make us.

Did you ever know of a genius whose eating habits, for instance, were not peculiar to himself? If he be but a fledgling genius, people call him "cranky;" or if fully-winged and widely-named, they call him "eccentric." Wrong, all wrong. Genius has been defined as *"an excess of normality."* It *is* just that—the quintessence of our common instincts, motives and desires, brought to the boiling-point. Mediocrity would not be bound if it knew how to break the fetters; Genius will not be bound because it does know how. And most of us secretly long to do the very things we condemn in the man who dares. Next to the child, may the genius set copy for the race. His script may not always be stupidly regular—but oh how graceful, how lordly are his capitals!

Did you ever observe that a weather-vane is the only thing the wind can't buffet? Its reward for daring to appear "flighty." But a weather-vane can't be upset, either. And a great soul needs fixity no less than a small soul needs mobility. We cannot be sane until we are symmetrical.

Now for a ray of sunshine. A "bad habit" is a good thing— *to outgrow.* Restriction is to the soul what trellis is to the morning-glory; a necessary support while climbing. The only way to escape it is to transcend it—not to fret over it or demand its destruction. The existence of anything sufficiently proves its beneficence; it is the *persistence* of the *same* thing that finally enthralls us. Things were made to use, then forget; but men abuse—then remember.

Conclude you ere now that I am a Freethinker? Not so, ineradicably not so. Freedom I have won—yet Freethinker am I not. Love I live in—yet Freelover am I not. I am *nothing which I can define.*

A Freelover has been denominated elsewhere.

A Freethinker is a rash youth that smashes guide-posts unread, without having brought his own chart and compass. The blazings on a forest path grow dim and dark with time; thus has superstition cast obloquy on the keen edge of Spirit. But if you are wise, you will look for the way-marks rather than the mould.

There are two means to darken a window; shade inside, shutter outside. The Freethinker has smashed into bits—boastful bits—the shutters of race-prejudice. But the *blind of his own mentality* is still down, and he mistakes the faint glow suffusing his understanding for the clear white light of the noonday sun.

He alone is free who is unconscious that fetters exist—for himself or anybody else. Freedom laughs at labels—the tags we wear mark rather our destination than our condition. As soon as a parcel gets anywhere, you take the tag off.

Now proportion is a question of perspective—you can't see much of the horizon through that ill-plumbed knot-hole of proximity. Habitude is a listless settling into the somnolence that surrounds us. Freedom is a mighty soaring into the sunlight that shines above us.

This is a province of the Conquest Fast—to give you the *freedom of far-sightedness.*

Freedom is an awful thing. Glorious, yet awful. To stand absolutely alone in the Universe; to watch, from your skyline-vantage, what people and things bound you to earth sink forever in the abyss of bondage; to stifle the sob and press back the tear; to lean like a child on the breast of Nature, and stretch out your hand for the Hand of God; this is the silent meeting of anguish and rapture, this is the vicarious At-one-ment.

Few souls are strong enough, brave enough, sane enough. But the one soul in a thousand who is ready for the Conquest Fast is worth more than all the rest. That consciousness is sufficient recompense for the heart's blood wherewith I write this book. For the only indelible writing has been traced by the writer in his own heart's blood.

The Conquest Fast makes you free in more ways than I can mention here. I have witnessed the prosecution of several. And in each case, a complete change in life-habits was the result. Your thinking, your feeling, your believing, your desiring, your planning, your hoping, your loving, *should* be your own after the Fast. It is safe to say they were not your own before the Fast.

The most vital change is usually the entire readjustment of eating-habits. And no more vital change could be effected for the salvation of the race.

Nowhere are men more hopelessly human than as they herd miserably together three times a day to get the money's worth of their board bill. *Natural beings eat alone.* They answer the call of Hunger—but they don't sit around waiting for it. They have no regular meal-hours, regularity being the cruel lash plied by the hand of a blind civilization. They don't gossip, find fault, read newspapers or complain of the food—hence are strangers to dyspepsia. They don't invoke the blessing of an all-wise Deity on such stupidly iniquitous fare as calf's brains, dumplings and brandy sauce. They don't gulp down the first helping for fear there won't be enough of the same for a second. They don't watch their neighbors when the pie is passed, to see who gets the biggest piece.

They don't do a hundred and one things that make men most ridiculous of the absurd in the way men eat. Ever notice how cross most husbands get if their wives don't sit at the table with them? She needn't eat—only preside at her lord's festal board. Heaven only knows why—unless to furnish additional proof that men *are* more unreasonable than women.

No, I do not agree with Charlotte Perkins Gilman in her claim that a home and a prison are identical. Not at all—for in a prison you're relieved of responsibility.

The remedy for prison-like homes is not *communism*—but *individualism*. When every member of the family has the same personal freedom he would have if there were no family—then will home begin to be home.

Valuable secret for wives free. How to Keep a Husband Home Nights. *"Open the door wide and prop it open."* The reason for propping it open is that he'll be back presently. That is, if he loves you. If he doesn't, you shouldn't want him back. Moreover, in case you are gracious enough—or wise enough—to give him a good-bye kiss as he passes out into the night, I prophesy he'll return before the shops are closed—purpose to bring you some flowers or sweets. Men are so contrary— so transparently contrary! If only they were as child-like in the ways they should be as they are in the way they shouldn't!

How we do wander away from the Fast.

We mustn't philosophize a bit more—in this chapter.

Eating should be either a festival or a sacrament—both if you can make it so. I think of all the lessons taught me through the Conquest Fast none has proved so continuously, so cumulatively helpful as this. We should eat as animals—or as gods. *Not as men.* Speaking metaphysically, our attitude should be either subconscious or superconscious, instead of grossly objective as it usually is. In short, we should *feel* with both body and soul; but not think with the brain. Here again, as in so many instances, the jar and the whirr of mere mental machinery has diverted us from the just enjoyment of our bodily senses, while deafening us to the finer appeal of our soul-sensibilities.   ,

Brain may re-enforce Instinct in this far: To guarantee the wholesomeness of every food set before you. Brain should then

retire—*without questioning the digestibility* of a single morsel.
Let Hunger enjoy, undisturbed.

By "festival" I do not mean sociability.

By "sacrament" I do not mean solemnity.

I can eat in a restaurant—if none of my friends are there.
And when I've worked hard, thus earning a good dinner, that's
where I go instead of to my cupboard. People who always prepare their own food get morbid on the subject.

But to observe meal-time as a sacrament, I must be utterly
alone—free of all personal vibrations. Which again contradicts
custom, all the church communicants gathering to commemorate
the Holy Supper. A sacrament can never be a commemoration;
ideals are sacred—but their ashes are earthy.

No "family table" any more?

Yes—if you have found who your family really are. There
are just three in my family circle—Nature, God and I. And our
family name is Love. We seldom have company at all—so few
people know our real name and residence. When mere humans
do come upon us by accident at meal-time, we always shudder—
We Three. Because they disrupt the serenity of the atmosphere
with their harsh echoes of civilization.

Do not call this churlishness. If all the race would let me
love it, I should never need to leave it. But in order to realize
that Love is the only thing worth while, one must first have suffered
a thousand eons. So we can only wait till the world grows tender.

Yearn and wait, in silence.

FASTING FOR POWER

CHAPTER IV.

Success is what the world pays a man for discovering and developing himself.

During the process of self-certifying, Providence kindly withholds this fact from him. Because if he knew it, he would be forever trying to sell the gold-mine unworked instead of exploring it with his own pick-axe. Indeed he might be tempted to salt it into the bargain.

I have not as yet developed myself—I have discovered myself. I know what's there. And I am quite willing for the world not to know, until my title be clearly established and my treasures safely stored. Because the world would certainly fetch its clumsy tools and attempt to dig. The world is always waiting to work the other fellow's mine. You see it hasn't found its own.

For Self-discovery I know nothing to take the place of the Conquest Fast. As an initial motive for self-development and a swift means thereto, it is also unequalled. *We cannot know ourselves until we get away from our surroundings.* Because most of us are but bits of polished wood reflecting faintly the sallow lights about us; instead of glowing firebrands kindled direct from the sun-glass of Truth above us.

Only the summit-vision can reveal the smallness of the world and the greatness of a human soul.

We are not, as a noted editor would always remind us, mere ants on the seashore or corals in the reef. We are partakers of Omnipotence. Undreamed-of powers are within us, possibilities around us. But sloth and fear, precedent and custom, ignorance and inertia, envy and interference crowd as terrifying phantoms between us and our opportunities.

Indeed most men fail to see their larger possibilities while watching too anxiously their smaller possessions. The Infinite is the realm of the potential. And you must look skyward to discern your own greatness.

To be powerful is to be in perfect command of all your faculties, at a given time, in a given place, under a given condition, for a given purpose.

Let us begin with strength of body.

We observe in the first place that fat and force are mutually exclusive. Louis Kuhne, the German Naturist, has shown convincingly that a fat man is a sick man. His excessively vital temperament may make him appear stronger than the man of nerve and sinew. But he can't do the work of his lithe brother, nor stand the strain, nor combat the disease that always threatens a successful man. Now nothing but a long Fast will prove to you *how little food you require* for the actual needs of the body. Not more than a third of what most men eat. With an increased enjoyment moreover and a constant feeling of buoyancy as delightful as it is unusual.

Every ounce of food taken in excess of hunger means so much dissipated energy. Take that same force from your stomach and put it into your business—both stomach and business will improve. A brain-worker is seldom really hungry unless he takes regular exercise at a gymnasium. He can eat a lot if he exercises a lot. But what's the use? To eat less and also exercise less comes to the same end. With a saving of time, money, thought and vitality.

A gymnasium is almost as unnatural as a church or a drugstore. All three are needless if the life-habits be right; eating, clothing, sleeping, bathing, working, resting, playing, thinking and loving. I know prominent systems of Physical Culture whose chief excuse for violent exercise is to create an equally violent appetite. Hunger can't be created—it comes of itself. All it asks of you is to wait for it—then satisfy it—then stop. You lose power if you treat it any other way.

Fatigue, or lack of endurance, is a common besetment of the business man. Weariness never indicates food—but always sleep. On the twenty-fourth day of my long Fast I took a tramp through the West Virginia Hills with a party of friends. Every one had eaten at least fifty meals since I had tasted food.   And at the close of the day I was as fresh as any.   I found repeatedly that *what seemed to be fatigue was only some remnant of undigested food* still lurking in my system.   A few eliminative measures quite refreshed me.

If every brain-worker were to spend half the noon-hour— or all of it in case he takes breakfast—in a quiet room apart, with eyes closed, body in repose, mentality suspended, breath rhythmic and regular; that afternoon ennui would all disappear.

Power is not generated in the stomach.   *You can never eat to get strong.*   A man's ability to do comes through his heart, his lungs, his brain and his soul.   The soul needs no material nourishment, the brain next to none, and the heart and lungs so little as scarcely to be reckoned.   Physical strength lies all in the breath, mental strength all in the brain, spiritual strength all in the soul.

Physiologists have always likened the human machine to an engine.   They have told us we must stoke the stomach about so often with a generous assortment of fuel—else the boiler would lose its enthusiasm.   The human machine is in reality a giant *dynamo.*   And you don't need much of a wood-pile or coal-yard to keep electricity going.

Before considering the brain phase, let us define power in its human application.

Power is the dynamic perception of possibilities.

He alone is powerful who can first see what to do—then do it.   Alertness of brain, steadiness of nerve, vigor of body, courage of soul; not one of these elements may be lacking.   Now no man can think and digest at the same time; notwithstanding the fact that many business deals are arranged over a specially elaborate luncheon.   And every day of a long Fast you will find your brain growing clearer.   Keenness of discernment, depth of insight, quickness of decision, breadth of vision, finality of judgment; all this you possess as never before.

Personally, a single morsel of food inhibits my creative work for the rest of the day.   I can do executive work in the afternoon. But only before the late breakfast at eleven or twelve, can I focus on a point or think to a hair-line.

The Conquest Fast removes from your brain your own faulty judgments and the still faultier opinions of your friends. It helps you see over, under, through and beyond a subject, with the power of an X-ray and the accuracy of a Goerz lens. Confusion of ideas is a condition of the past. You grasp *all of one idea* instead of *pieces of many*. And on the breadth of this basis you can act with confidence.

Progress is a combination of *judicial attitude* with *intuitive action*. You must be able to see all sides of the question at once— then act with the freedom of spontaneity and the courage of conviction. This means both brilliancy of brain and illumination of soul. Few people have either. Almost nobody has both together. But if it's possible for you to realize this double boon, the Conquest Fast will give it to you.

The initiation of originality is a basic element in human power. This also the Fast will enhance—perhaps awaken for the first. Great ideas are born in souls not content to adopt small imitations. And a soul strong enough to take an extreme Fast in defiance of race-belief voluntarily puts itself in touch with Creativity.

God is more dreamer than thinker, more lover than both. And when God sees in one individual a soul that dare dream for itself, with a brain that dare think for itself and a will that dare act for itself—God loves that being peculiarly, blessing it in some special sense.

There is no enduring power save transcendence of soul. Money tarnishes, fame withers, friendship wanes, beauty fades, success palls and worlds end in dust. But to the soul that can leave the mortal when it chooses, sustaining itself on air, water, light, faith and love—there are no limitations, no disappointments, no doubts, no fears, no disabilities, no misunderstandings, no tremors whatsoever.

Truth is as clear as the sky above, destiny as bright as the noonday sun, and life as sweet as the nurturing breast of the Universal Mother.

Crowning all comes a consciousness of Omnipotence; that makes of this world a little play-room, of mortal possessions a box of toys, of the human race a handful of tin soldiers; and of you owner of the nursery, disposer of the toys, Commander of the host.

FASTING FOR BEAUTY

CHAPTER V.

Beauty is a long story—ask any woman.

But this is a short chapter—short enough for any man.

Experiment writes essays; Experience writes epigrams.

Not that I am adept in boudoir legerdemain. Only a general averment anent authorcraft.

Beauty is soul-deep.

I think even a man will agree to this. At least if he has ever had a sweetheart whose eyes answered the light in his own.

But beauty is more than soulfulness. You can't cure a muddy complexion with a smile, or fill out hollows by means of a tranquil mind. Beauty is *too natural to be occult*. What desirable thing isn't? Nature made beauty paramount with health. You can't separate them. And any woman content to be other than beautiful is other than wholesome.

Take for instance Dress Reform. The garb it whacks out may be a consolation to the lady that wears it—no woman would wear it—but it's an eyesore to everybody else. Sackcloth and ashes go together. And there's no place on a sackcloth gown for the rose of your admiration. You think at once of the ash-barrel. Indeed that's where all reformers belong—in the ash-barrel. I stopped being a reformer just in time to escape it. I'm glad—for the sake of the ash-barrel. It hadn't hurt anybody.

I don't recall the artist's definition of beauty. But in general I believe human beauty to be made up of seven elements; Form, Color, Texture, Posture, Proportion, Expression, Animation.

Now the secret of beauty, thus defined, is perfect metabolism. I mean physiologically, of course. And with the possible exception of Proportion, every one of these seven elements is enhanced, or restored to its pristine perfection, by the regenerative power of the Conquest Fast.

Fasting won't work miracles. Only the plastic surgeon or the advertising dermatologist can do that. Fasting won't rectify crooked noses, or melt moles from the cheek, or make the windows of the soul look inviting while the blinds are still down. The blinds go up though during the Fast, don't they? I forgot. But every bit of beauty you're entitled to as the just fruition of your past lives, the Conquest Fast will give you.

Take Form.

Suppose you weigh too much. When you come to regain the weight lost through the Fast, you will stop short of the excess. I was ten pounds overweight before my Fast. After it I was normal. Or if you lack flesh, you will put it on. By the same renewal of the powers of assimilation. In short, inequalities will be leveled, and symmetry ensue.

Take Color.

The delicacy of tint that will mantle your face can be approached by nothing save the memory of childhood. Skin blemishes will disappear. Extreme redness or whiteness will be modified. Even enlarged pores will subside. I'm not talking poetry now. Beauty is poetic. But every woman knows that the average beauty stunt is prosiest of the prosy.

Take Texture.

Did you ever compare the foreheads of a prize-fighter and a poet? Not alone in form and contour, but equally in the texture of the skin is the difference manifest. The prize-fighter lives on beefsteak and "sinkers"; the poet on—well, mostly air and optimism. Of course if he's a magazine poet, he will sometimes be invited out to dine, and occasionally receive a cheque. But we're speaking now of real poets, the kind the world isn't ready for till they die. The fibre of your flesh will refine noticeably, even before you finish the Fast, and in the end it will be smooth as the petal of a rose-bud.

Take Posture.

Ever observe how many people sag in the middle? This chronic collaption may be traced to two causes; too much dinner and not enough self-respect. The Conquest Fast subtracts the dinner and adds the self-respect.

Take Expression.

Which includes the sparkle in the eye, the blush on the cheek, the smile about the lips, in a word the ensemble of the countenance. Health brings Hope. And only Hope can illume the human face with an aura angelic.

Take Animation.

By this I mean sensitivity, responsiveness, feeling. Most people are unattractive because moribund. You can't beautify the pallor of a corpse in the making. Put Life into the human body, Love into the human heart, Light into the human soul:— and lo, a being of beauty arises in the majesty of newly awakened Selfhood. Life, Light and Love—this exactly sums the Conquest Fast.

That's all.

I said it would be short, didn't I?

Surely in one chapter I should be kind to you.

P. S. You won't be conspicuously beautiful *while* you're fasting—not till afterwards. So don't be haunting the mirror. Lest the mirror haunt you.

FASTING FOR FAITH

CHAPTER VI.

We love only verities; we fear only phantoms.

So if we could everywhere see the real through the shadow, we should always love and never fear.

Faith is the focus of our verity-vision.

And the nicety of its adjustment determines our whole outlook on life.

Some souls are far-sighted—but blind to the things adjacent. More souls are near-sighted—but blind to the things beyond. While the majority of souls are afflicted with moral astigmatism. The only cure for which, as you know, being to improve the general health.

Occasionally some really sane soul visits this planet, and proceeds to apprehend realities both near and far. Forthwith is that soul set upon by the hordes of the half-blind, who demand that it renounce *either* its earth-vision *or* its heaven-vision and become as one of them. If it cannot or will not, they call it fool, knave or lunatic, crucify it if they dare, ostracize it in any event, then settle back into their stupid daze with the consciousness of duty well done. This is the penalty for having a faith *both religious and scientific.* But it's worth it. With both God and Nature back of you, men can't avail against you to any considerable degree.

The faith that proves sees equally well with eyes open or eyes closed. It makes fact the foundation of its structure, but builds its tower out of imagination. Needless to say, it keeps its supplies in the cellar, while locating its study in the observatory.

Faith is usually an owl—it sees best by night.

While Reason is usually a chicken—it runs to roost at dusk. What the world needs is a Luther Burbank of Metaphysics, to cross the species and produce a creature not a cripple either by day or by night.

The tendency of modern thought is to reject faith altogether. If it does, modern man dies. He who robs a soul of its faith is both marauder and murderer; since no soul can flourish long in that arctic midnight of Doubt. *Better a thousand times to trust Error than to doubt Truth.* It is the act of believing, not the object of belief, that makes man courageous for doing. Humans have won great victories in the name of Zeus, and of Allah, and of Jehovah. Yet Zeus, Allah and Jehovah are none of them God. Faith but lifts us a little way out of the darkness that envelopes us. If it be but a little way, let us be glad for that—not fretful that the light fails of being perfect.

Almost invariably those who reject the letter of the Bible lose also its spirit. Because the Book of books records much that is human superstition, the Freethinker denies therein more that is divine Truth. Omniscience reveals to man only so much as man is ready for. So our light should be greater, rather than less, in comparison with the early seers and apostles. But they had the *attitude of belief*—we have the attitude of doubt. And while credence is not credulity, it is farther removed from the habit of denial.

Knowledge is the father and Faith the mother of Enthusiasm. Enthusiasm can't be born without Knowledge; but only Faith can rear it. You try to achieve some great purpose apart from the leadership of Enthusiasm—then see where you end.

Faith, like all other realities, is much misunderstood and maligned. For instance, Faith without works is not "dead." It's imaginary. It never existed. You can't keep Faith torpid any more than you can sunlight. It is the very essence of energy. And the piously pale brethren who never mingle with the world because they're so busy exercising their faith—they have a dead faith and are too numb to know it. A live one wouldn't stay with them ten seconds. For fear of getting a fatal chill.

Faith moreover is not an occult phantasm. It's natural, it's human, it's whole-souled and warm-hearted. I used to be a chronic disputer, an inveterate denier. I doubted everybody and everything. Myself particularly. Was I human? Far from it. I looked like a ghost, acted like a paralytic, and felt like a miserable memory. Today I believe in everybody and everything. Myself particularly. And I'm a regular dynamo of energy.

Believing is achieving. And there is nothing so deadening as to lose the beautiful faith of our childhood; faith in people, faith in the future, faith in food, faith in sleep, faith in play, faith in work—yes, and faith in fairies, dreams, visions. The way of life is a belt-line, whose beginning and end is childhood. You haven't seen it all till you've been clear around.

Why and how do we lose our faith? Because we do not think, feel and act for ourselves. That's all. In every crisis of life, comes the guiding whisper of Instinct, Intuition, Inspiration, or some other voice of the soul. But the din of the world without has deafened us, the shadow of appearance has blinded us, the advice of false friends has dissuaded us. Next time the voice sounds weaker. Presently it is still. Then has doubt settled into despair. We have bartered the certitude of soul God gave us for the maze of mind offered by men.

Now, briefly, what is the office of the Conquest Fast? Just this. *To establish beyond peradventure* the three kinds of faith I deem most vital; *faith in Nature, faith in Self, faith in God.*

Faith in Nature ensures health.

Faith in Self ensures success.

Faith in God ensures abiding peace.

What more can we ask? What more do we need? Just how the Fast operates to this end I have not space to describe here. But how it operated on at least one human being you will find recorded at the close of this book, under the heading—"A Declaration of Faith." Most of these beliefs of mine developed directly or indirectly as a result of the long Fast. I wouldn't have the same set come to you for anything—if our minds were just alike, I'm sure we'd both be uncomfortable. Let us say better beliefs will be yours—I shan't feel the least bit envious.

May your faith also grow till it spans earth and sea and sky, comprehending all that in them is. Then may it emerge from the constriction of the tangible, to lay hold everlastingly on the sublime potentials in the keeping of the Unseen.

FASTING FOR COURAGE.

CHAPTER VII.

A good man may have the courage of his convictions—only a great man has the courage of his intuitions.

We wear convictions; we live intuitions.

Convictions are mostly second-hand, shop-worn, and moth-eaten. We either inherit them from our ancestors or borrow them from our neighbors. And as our neighbors and ancestors had borrowed them before us, nobody knows whom they really fitted in the first place. He wouldn't own them now anyway—they've sagged all out of shape, been patched and pinned and puckered, dyed a dozen different shades in as many spots; in short are ready for the rag-bag generally.

An entire outfit of respectable convictions is called a reputation—you find this ensemble at a sewing society or a church festival. It won't be at the same clacque twice though,—it never survives one. Then people struggle to refurbish it. It only looks worse. Never try to scrub the stains off a soiled reputation—you'll tear holes in it. If they won't wear off in time—get a new reputation, one that will wash. Then stay where the soot doesn't gather. Which means where nobody lives.

I took my Conquest Fast in the midst of a college community. Nobody lives there. It's true they're generally nobodies—but none of them live.

A college community is a quarantine of unfortunates, afflicted mostly with paralysis of the heart, goose-flesh of the conscience, and hyperkinesis of the tongue. Nothing will cure these ailments but a sojourn in the sanitarium of Life. And this the classicist is always averse to.

I find I'm getting a trifle sarcastic along in here. Some of the chapters though are extra solemn; while a sentiment here and there may seem sweet to you. So if you mix them all together, you should get an average of measurable temperateness.

Nothing is so conducive to courage as to controvert and set at nought a fixed race-belief. Do you know anything the race believes in more than in eating?

Study the lives of the world's great men.

See how uniformly they were dominated by some one bold idea that the world then called unreasonable and unattainable. Science, invention, music, art, literature, therapeutics—even religion; these have all been enriched most largely by men considered mad during their lifetime.

Healing, for example, has been most promoted by pioneers outside the regular school. I have but to mention these names: Hahnemann, Ling, Kneipp, Kuhne, Lahmann, Schroth, Rikli, Just, Weltmer, Babbitt, Macfadden, Still, Wilmans, Eddy;—the list is endless. These benefactors of the race had the courage that comes from an *individual, cumulative and practicable ideal.* The greatest of them being Jesus the Nazarene.

They never saw the impotent panic of the world that witnessed their heresy; they saw Truth and Truth was enough. Deify the world and it damns you; damn it and it deifies you. The self-conscious soul never asks "Can I measure up to men's expectations?" Rather, "Must I measure down to them?" And all compromise is defeat.

Every soul that dares to be true to itself has passed through Gethsemane and faces Golgotha. If the world does not tear its flesh with spikes that spill its blood on the cross, it is because the spewings of anathema and the thorns of persecution are more subtly cruel. Think you then that courage is a possession to be underestimated?

To return to my Fast amidst the academicians.

For the purpose of heightening its effect, I made the conditions as hard as possible; the subsequent joy of conquest being proportionally vivid.

I walked the streets while the town gossiped. I worked instead of rested, giving lectures at a Summer School then in progress. I projected myself into all sorts of hostile vibrations from people who did not understand and did not want to. By the time the thirty days were over, I had courage enough to defy a thousand worlds if need be, in the attaining of my ideal. Not that the attitude of defiance is a desirable one. But sometimes you have to take it to avoid being demolished. A very sensitive soul has to protect itself from assaults. Often by personal peculiarities that tend to repel people, better by triumphs of successful activity that tend to awe them. If you be such a soul, cultivate *postivity* at any cost. Forget your visions for a while, and get down to business.

Courage is chiefly subjective in motive. So is the Conquest Fast.

Courage is chiefly objective in method. So is the Conquest Fast.

In the face of misfortune, a strong man weeps while a weak woman smiles. Why? Because the woman's courage lies in her soul, the man's in his brain and body. At the desertion of the tangible, naturally the woman rises to meet the emergency. Moreover then, and then only, is she thoroughly practical—when her soul takes command. *That human is courageous who never sees the limitations of the mortal, but always the potentials of the eternal.*

Examples; The somnambule safely skirting a six-inch ledge three stories above the ground (I know personally of such cases); the inebriate falling into fire, water and a variety of perils, yet coming forth unscathed; the cripple aroused by the call of "Fire!" to spontaneous effort that sends his crutches flying and his stiffened body now straight and strong, to a place of security; the fragile mother braving ominous dangers and surmounting impassable obstacles in order to protect or advance her offspring.

All these derive their courage from momentary *blindness to the objective.* God has told them they can! So for the time they forget how the world says they can't.

God will tell *you,* "You can!"

No matter what—*You can.*

If you want to know how and why and where, let your senses be refined for receptivity through the Conquest Fast.

FASTING FOR POISE

CHAPTER VIII.

The most magnificent spectacle I ever saw was a storm in the Alps.

We had climbed above the cloud-line. Above the verdure-line also—since clouds gather always and only in the region of mortality. The storm broke suddenly, a way storms have in the higher altitudes. On the lowlands, one has time to seek shelter. But every step upward is a step away from surety.

Through the darkening mist, we could just discern the thatched Swiss village far below; and the people hurrying to house their fragile possessions. Little children ran crying to their mothers; children of a larger growth followed not a long way behind. Even the Swiss kine, those models of mute endurance, paused in their grazing and stood as if awestruck in the face of the heavens' upheaval.

Here and there a mountain-peak was still lit with celestial splendor. But its neighbor, opposite and below, was plunged in the gloom of midnight. Nothing can be so impressive as the contrast between earth and sky when your vantage-vision penetrates both. All at once a blinding flash burst from the arsenal of the gods; swift on its trail of fire rolled their heavy artillery; completing the charge came shower after shower of melted missiles; and the fusillade was on.

Of all places over this earth, God and Nature make their tryst amid the Alpine fastnesses. There sky is clearer, sun is brighter, winds are fresher, waters are cooler, stars are closer;— and storms, when they come, are wilder. Everything is elemental; now tender as a dove, now savage as a tiger, but *always sincere.* Just as true lovers, when alone, bare their hearts and bodies to each each other, enduring not the least vestige of anything man-made between them; so here in the summit solitude blend God and Nature utterly, beautifully—terribly.

It is said that lightning strikes only decaying trees and diseased men. Whether or not this be so, it is certain that one must be very whole to smile in the face of an Alpine storm. And we pitied the villagers below.

But where we stood, all was sunshine—not the faintest streak of gray to tinge the transparent blue above us. The clouds might spend their impotent rage beneath us—we remained unscathed, untouched, unmoved, mere lookers-on. Meanwhile I was making an important discovery; that *a cloud always keeps its silver lining on the skyward side.* I think one has to stand himself above, before he ever observes this fact.

On the peak of the Cosmic Consciousness, storms never beat, misfortunes never settle, vicissitudes never venture, disasters never fall. To the soul that has yearned for solitude, ascended into silence, dared isolation—and triumphed, there appear no longer any mists of mortality. For that soul has climbed above the cloud-line.

Nothing matters.
I repeat; nothing matters.
But the only man who can safely say this is the man who brings things to pass. The yogi usually affirms it—and the average yogi better hadn't. The captain of industry almost never does—and he of all mortals needs to. In short, the phlegmatic temperament should learn how to hustle, the nervous temperament should learn how to rest. Not the proclivity we are born with promotes our growth toward symmetry; but the proclivity we create for ourselves. I am naturally keyed to the highest pitch of nervous activity—almost "hyperkinetic," the doctor would call it. Yet I can sink into a deeper repose than the most stolid individual I know. Because I am master first of myself, then of all the elements in the Universe I need to supplement myself.

Be a business man for the sake of your brain, be a Naturist for the sake of your body, be a mystic for the sake of your soul. If you are, you'll be the first whole human that ever lived.

Patience, Poise, Perspective; these are three conspicuous lacks of the average American.

We are not patient with ourselves or with others. We unduly lengthen our shortcomings. We magnify trifles and minify principles. We grasp at the shadow and lose the reality. We get rich by sundown and die by midnight to pay for it. We exalt the result of our action instead of exalting the action itself.

Impatience is the penalty for doing poor work.

Thoroughness is the one cure.

Poise is the balance-wheel of power. And God turns it. The most successful men are the ones who can smile at themselves for wanting to be successful. They get *on* in business because they know how to take a day *off* from business. It is the practice of a well-known financier to close his desk and run away, whenever the desk gets full of matters *too important to postpone.* To focus every faculty and fibre on one's work—then to forget it ever existed; this is the sane life. Most people are half-asleep by day and half-awake by night; they don't do anything all over. Mobility of soul is a rare and priceless accomplishment.

If we withdrew oftener from our treadmill-round, we should observe we're not getting anywhere. In order for our work, our creed, our aspiration to expand, we must be larger than them all, must see beyond them, must live above them.

Take the Vegetarians, for instance—poor, woe-begone creatures. They could be rendering us a two-fold service, if they would occupy themselves converting the mosquitoes. I'm sure both the hygienic and ethical arguments of Vegetarianism would particularly appeal to a mosquito. And we should get a momentary rest. I know an honored Vegetarian whose one joy in meeting strangers seems to be to air his boast, "I haven't tasted meat for twenty years." So? I can go you one better. I haven't tasted angle-worms since I was a robin-redbreast, ten million years ago. But I have something better to do than parade Broadway with my back placarded to that effect.

Let me remark in passing that I believe in a non-meat diet. But I wear neither tag nor blinders.

Because my belief marks the limits of my brain, shall I say to my soul, "Thus far—and no further"?

Patience, poise, perspective;—and what of the Conquest Fast?

I can't tell you. There are no words.

Words may paint shadows—only feelings can sense realities.

But if you will gaze steadfastly into the heavens for days and nights without interruption, you shall realize for yourself. In the other books on Fasting I have asked you to read, you find no mention of this phase. If you study, however, the lives of Buddha, Jesus, and a few other unimpeachable Messiahs, the vision of the hill-top will explain itself. These all fasted, first for the sake of the soul. So did I. So may you.

The simple act of omitting breakfast regularly, and taking a long walk instead, will conduce to patience, poise, and perspective. Especially if you rise with the sun. Some subtle magnetism, some ethereal elixir seems to charge the early morning air; before the world is astir and the jarring vibrations from multitudes of un-attuned mortals have once more resumed their daily jangle. Day-dreams that come true awake with the dawn.

But if you want to see the world from a new angle alto-gether; to feel Truth with a sense of finality; to apportion things large and small their real evaluation; to distinguish between the immortal soul of you and its earthly facilities of mind and body; to realize the nothingness of time and the allness of Eternity; to abide unperturbed while nations war, empires fall, and worlds pass away;—then go on the mountain or beside the sea, and achieve *your* Conquest Fast.

FASTING FOR VIRTUE

CHAPTER IX.

This chapter is specially recommended to clergymen, "high livers," and other erring ones addicted to chicken dinner on Sunday.

There's nothing inherently vicious about the chicken—Nature made it. But there is in the trimmings—a French chef made them.

Paris vice is the post-prandium to Paris viands.

London vice to London viands, Berlin vice to Berlin viands, New York vice to New York viands. Since it is no more unrighteous to be a volatile Frenchman than to be a beefy Englishman, a dense German, or a neurotic American.

I ask not if a man be holy—I ask if he be whole. And these one-sided racialists are none of them whole.

Wholeness presupposes and ensures holiness. Since vice is a matter, not of moral depravity, but of physical and mental excess or deficiency. The Conquest Fast reduces this excess and reveals this deficiency. Herein is it advisable for those also who pride themselves on being "exemplary"—they lack good red blood and riot in bad blue thought. Incidentally I may observe you can't "set" a good example—it isn't stationary.

Speaking of good red blood. It has been a time-honored fallacy of both Physiology and Theology that white corpuscles made pure blood. Redundant perhaps to say "time-honored fallacy"—since fallacies are about the only things time honors anyway. In matters of morals especially has the anaemic been mistaken for the virtuous, and the ruddy for the vicious. We now know—at least a few of us do—that the more red corpuscles the better the blood; and the redder they are the purer it is. Quality counts—not color. For white corpuscles are but disease-clots.

The whitest part of the lily is not the mother-part. Wholly encircled by white, as passion always should be, it enters on a deeper hue when once it finds its heart. Prudery wears lilies—to appear pure; Love, being pure, may wear the roses that symbolize power. I like them best together though—roses and lilies in the same vase. My Sweetheart does too. Even to mention one's sweetheart to others is almost sacrilege. Certainly to describe her is to defame her. You may be glad you are reading instead of listening. Because then—unless you are one of the few rare souls that understand—I should hardly feel like speaking of Love at all.

Only Love prizes equally roses and lilies.

Only lovers therefore will sense my meaning in this chapter.

It is worse to be so good you can't be bad, than so bad you won't be good.

If saints are as valuable as sinners, why should saints spend their lives saving sinners?

A sinner is a man who can't live without loving; a reformer is a man who can't love at all.

Now I've done it. Henceforth am I ostracized by the respectable and excommunicated by the pious. A terrible fate— but shared by all the great souls that have ever lived.

There are compensations though. For instance, I shan't get any more fishy handshakes.

Understand, I am neither arraigning virtue nor defending vice.

Both defense and arraignment imply counter-charge. And I never argue. We argue solely to convince ourselves. Since assured of myself, I have outgrown disputation.

My neighbor's virtue or vice is none of my business—until he asks me to make it so. But when my own virtue is condemned as vice and vice extolled as virtue, it's in order for me to say a word. This has often happened.. Hence several words.

First let us define "sin."

Sin is the temporary thwarting of the soul by forces outside itself. "Saving souls" is therefore an absurdity.

Salvation is *the soul's assumption of its right to rule*—no more, no less. He therefore is a savior who can help the soul best, quickest and fullest to express itself.

I recognize that what the church calls sin does thwart the soul. But only temporarily. And it is *less of an evil to be thwarted than to be throttled.* Any expression is better than all repression. Indeed the greatest mistake proves to be the greatest lesson in disguise. If the soul *knew* itself it *would not sin;* if it *trusted* itself it *could* not sin.

Theology actually causes much of the sin it would remedy— by teaching the soul to fear itself instead of to know and trust. Ignorant of realities and terrified by symptoms, both Medicine and Theology have dosed the sufferer with germicides and antipyretics. Result to body and soul; congestion, stagnation, death. This because we take the temperature and look at the tongue, rather than learn wherein Nature has been violated. If souls were as apprehensive of enteric fever as they are of eczema, the death-rate of souls would be cut in two.

It is almost never justifiable to *remain* a "sinner;" it is almost always justifiable to *become* a sinner. Better love the wrong thing than not to love at all—but next time, love the right thing. You see there's hardly anybody to tell us what the right thing is. So we seldom know until, alone and forsaken, we have somehow stumbled on it for ourselves.

No—not alone, and not forsaken. God was with us through the sin that men condemned. Indeed, that is why they condemned —because God had left their hearts to comfort ours.

Anything is sin that sounds louder than the voice of your own soul. It may be sinful for you to hear a sermon, or join in prayer;—if the sermon and the prayer represent some childish notion of Deity that you have outgrown.

Now the soul has four principal mediums of communication; *instinct, intuition, inspiration,* and *revelation.* To violate any one of these is to sin. Instinct is what makes us good animals—or would if we would let it. But the instinct in most of us is dead— it isn't "nice" to be like animals. I often wish the beasts of the field and the birds of the air could laugh—how they would ridicule men! No they wouldn't either; it takes a man to be uncharitable —animals don't know how.

No wonder men aren't in possession of themselves. They attribute to the animals all their bad qualities and to the gods all their good ones. I think both animals and gods would be improved by a judicious interchange. Indeed the old heathen gods, with their half-human grotesqueness, were often nearer Truth than our modern Deities of glossy raiment and wooden hearts.

I have treated somewhat on this matter of instinct in another chapter. Let me merely say in passing that *the violation of instinct is the beginning of all vice.* It is just as truly a crime to wear a tight shoe or to eat when not hungry as to murder a fellow-man. Not so much of a crime, of course. Many a temperance reformer is a worse drunkard than the rum victim he condemns. He is a *food-inebriate.* He habitually stuffs himself on viands that vitiate every atom of his being. Equally with the drunkard is he a slave to the senses—and on top of that a hypocrite. Any minister who *must have* his cigar knows less real religion than the weed he smokes.

Before proceeding further, let me give you my idea of virtue.

Virtue consists in the utmost expression of the divine through the natural.

Not through the human—since the human is seldom the natural. Seldom therefore the divine, there being no distinction. I am not moral. Neither am I immoral. I am *unmoral*—like both animals and angels. I do not defend or condone wanton wickedness. The man who entices a virgin to corruption should pay the severest penalty. But the man who *loves* a virgin and is loved of her—no law need they to authorize what God has implanted.

In short, *the abandon of unmorality is as desirable as the wantonness of immorality is deplorable.*

Here again I am quite willing to stand alone. It's rather exhilarating when you get used to it—nothing human to shut off the hills, the sun, and the stars.

To be famous, one must do what others cannot.

To be infamous, one must do what others dare not. Count me with the few great souls that *must do both*.

We're a long time getting to the Conquest Fast.

But we couldn't come cross-lots, because there were some things of interest I wanted to point out along the path we took.

Dr. Edward Hooker Dewey, to whom I have already referred, has written another book, a sequel to his first. In this he shows how Fasting may be made an almost infallible cure for Chronic Alcoholism. If you care to study further the relation of food to virtue and to vice, you should by all means get this book.

The point is simply this.

During the Conquest Fast, *one's taste for everything unnatural wholly disappears.* Liquors, tobacco, spiced foods, tight clothing, perfervid literature, church worship, loveless passion, civilized habits;—these all go glimmering. Even so piquant a thing as a problem play ceases to appeal.

A problem play is an interrogation-point lost in the mud. And the problem is why the author forgot the soap. Which is irrelevant, but interesting.

The clue to race regeneration lies right here.

For ages, our moralists, theologians and reformers have mistaken human *encrustment* for human *integument.*

"Spirit is willing, but flesh is weak"? No. Flesh is not weak. Soul is impeded not by very flesh, but *by the externals that cumber flesh.* Clear your blood of wrong food, your lungs of wrong air, your brain of wrong thought, your nerves of wrong tremors, your heart of wrong fear, and your soul of wrong residue from all these other wrong things;—then see how absolutely right the whole world becomes.

The Conquest Fast won't transform a sinner into a god through the space of twenty, thirty or forty days. It takes eons of evolution to do that. And on this planet the process is but begun.

But it will hasten the end desired—perhaps help you skip an incarnation or two. There's no hurry though, time being purely imaginary. So if you'd rather "eat, drink and be merry" *all* the while, I haven't the least objection. *Once* in a while I like a sumptuous dinner too—and like it mighty well. We wouldn't be natural if we didn't. "Be a good animal"—that's Nature's first commandment, with promise.

FASTING FOR SPIRITUALITY

CHAPTER X.

I used to get the headache whenever I went to prayer-meeting.

A prayer-meeting is a place where you can substitute words for feelings without fear of detection.

Naturally I got the headache. Religion doesn't belong in the brain—it belongs in the heart. Starve your heart and stuff your brain—and you may expect moral vertigo. Even a doctor could prognosticate that much.

A sermon is mostly a dissection of Deity. And you can't dissect a thing till it's dead. Theology as a whole, is a postmortem examination on God. The form is all there, but somehow the soul is gone. A church is too musty for God to live in—God's very breath is freedom, God's life is sunlight. God is more animal than man. Whereas theologians are skimped as animals, and skewed even as men. God never taught in a theological seminary—*God was always too heterodox.* The only place God teaches is in the School of Nature. It is a boarding-school, and Nature provides most liberally for her wards. But the children prefer that hokey-pokey vendor named Orthodoxy. That's why they aren't hungry for their meals. It's why they're sallow, too— you can't make red blood out of any sort of sop.

I do not condemn a church service unqualifiedly. I have only three objections to it—the prayers, the hymns and the sermon. I believe in the kind of prayer that *says* nothing, *feels* everything —then *acts.* I believe in the song that thrills of itself from the throat of the lark, or the lover, or the woman just glorified by motherhood as she watches with the angels over her first babe. I believe in the sermon that a *silent life* makes most eloquent.

I do *not* believe in formal prayers.

I do *not* believe in paid choirs.

I do *not* believe in professional sermonizers. The world at large though needs these things—else it wouldn't tolerate them.

It needs Sunday observance—I need it myself. It needs the calm, the music, the flowers, the holy awe, the reflection and aspiration that distinguish the Day of Rest from the days and nights of turmoil. Sunday should be a synonym for saneness. Physically and psychologically we need just the change we get. Spiritually we need a change we do *not* get. If a man must sermonize, let him put on the overalls during the week. Let him toil and plan, and fail and starve, and sin and suffer and weep—*with Humanity*. *Then* let him tell how his faith has delivered him; and the people will throng the outer doors to hear him—he is now one of them. He has certified his message.

It is the Christlessness of the church that makes men irreligious.

Jesus the Nazarene was the sweetest, sanest, dearest soul that has yet come and gone on this planet. Jesus the Christ was, and is, the fullest embodiment of Deity yet revealed to men. But should he appear in the flesh to us, the church of to-day would brand Jesus the Nazarene a sinner and scout Jesus the Christ for an anarchist.

We none of us mean to crucify Truth—we are only beside ourselves with the fever of externalism. The same things that make us unnatural make us undivine. In the beginning, God resided happily in every human heart. But while Humanity was passing through the blind trance of Civilization, God grew weary waiting for something to do. So God stole away. When Humanity awoke, there was only God's outer garment left. And they call that religion—a form and a name. No man who *calls* himself theologian or metaphysician can truly heal the human soul. *Only Silence heals*—silent sympathy and silent knowledge.

Now we come to Spirituality—a possession almost as little understood and as much misunderstood as Love. Which is as strong as words can make it. Spirituality is *seldom found inside the church* and *never recognized outside*. Pseudo-spirituality is the curse of all organized religion. Let me mention a few brands—imitations very widely and successfully passed off as genuine.

Spirituality is *not Piety.*

They never go together, even. Spirit is Infinite Energy. Whereas the "pious" are confessedly impotent. Many a pious man is good—in spite of his religion. Good, but not spiritual. A corpse is always good.

Spirituality is *not Solemnity.*

Life is too serious to be solemn over. Even in a graveyard you may smell the flowers instead of reading the tombstones. Those on whom God smiles never frown back at God. Any god you *can* frown at is an idol. And idols are always sorrowful things.

Spirituality is *not Credulity.*

When you *know*, how can you cherish a blind belief? Spirituality is an all-pervading consciousness, that penetrates the unseen and assures the uncertain. A man may be religious—and ignorant. He cannot be spiritual—and ignorant.

Spirituality is *not Regularity.*

To pray regularly is to pray never. The security of small souls lies in regularity, that of great souls in spontaneity. Only a great soul can be spiritual—or spontaneous. Many a man who "hasn't missed church a single Sunday for twenty years" has missed God every Sunday for twenty years.

Spirituality is *not Loquacity.*

All the inspiration of Heaven you can put into three little words—"I love you." You don't even need words—just radiate it. When I meet people, I do not murmur "Pleased to know you." But I give them a smile and a handclasp that speak volumes—if they have learned the language of the heart; if they haven't, we must remain strangers anyway. Talk is the dissipation of the idle—work is the conservation of the spiritual. And they seldom unite.

Spirituality is *not Loyalty.*

How many a complaisant mortal has tried to excuse his inertness with some such sentiment as this "I never bother with these new-fangled religions—my father's God is good enough for me." Was your father's *life* good enough for you? For his life was but a miniature copy of his God. You may inherit your theology—it's mostly a matter of heirlooms. But you can't get spirituality that way—it's "made fresh every hour." No, I am not irreverent—spirituality is sweeter than any confection and more strengthening than the "staff of life."

Spirituality is *not Charity*.

Spirituality gives,—gives without stint. But of *itself*—not of its possessions. Moreover it never announces or recalls the fact. Can the river stop at any one point and say to the shore "I give you a pint to-day; be good and you may get a pint and a drop to-morrow"? The subtlest satisfaction in giving comes to him who leaves his name off the gift. The "anonymous" giver is surest of having his name recorded in Heaven.

Spirituality is *not Subtlety*.

There's nothing occult about it, nothing esoteric, theological, or even ethical. A bird can't flutter and fly at the same time; the occultist flutters since too feeble yet to fly. You can hear the flop of his wings and see the roll of his eyes—but you can't discern him getting anywhere. I call to mind a lecture given in New York not long since by a Theosophist of international fame. He was discoursing beautifully on the subject of "Auras"—pink, blue, red, white and yellow—with generous advice on how to dye our own the proper hue. Suddenly the stereopticon sputtered, gasped, flickered and gave up the ghost. Then you should have seen the aura of that venerable lecturer—it looked like a London fog hung up to dry in a Pittsburg smoke-house! After that I lost interest in his dyeing recipes.

Nor does Spirituality attend seances for the purpose of materializing itself to order. Spiritists cling pitifully to the personal, the tangible, the form of earth rather than the essence of the Eternal. Whether or not they prove their friends' immortality, they prove their own mortality. One example of the unsaneness of the occult. A certain well-known physician, deeply versed in eerie lore, asked me to come and see him shortly after my first book of poems appeared. He turned to the poem called "The Kiss," gave me a shocked and sorrowing look, and delivered himself somewhat in this wise—"Do you not fear you will be haunted forever by ten thousand evil spirits, each leering to see how you have glorified passion?" There was no answer— I only smiled. And yet my heart sank—how could he so misunderstand?

Spirituality is *not Fixity*.

The spiritual man is anchored to nothing save his own soul. Which makes him seem at times like a leaf tossed by the wind. Then the world decides he has "unsafe religious views." To *be everything* religiously is to *seem nothing* to your friends in the church. They have just so many labels stowed away by Custom in the pigeon-holes of their brain. And their only hope of understanding you is to make one of these price-tags fit. But Truth can't be ticketed—it grows more valuable every minute. So by the time the world has arrived at the symbol which appraises you—only your memory survives to be identified. *The heretics of to-day are the martyrs of to-morrow and saints of the day after.* Know then that to be termed heretic by the world, is to be foretold benefactor to the world.

Spirituality is *not Authority*.

It resides in no book, is limited by no creed, asks no church's support, and cares for no man's opinion. Spirituality is its own sanction. You cannot add to it by any revelation given another, you cannot take from it by any revelation denied another. It in itself is final—nothing without can make it more so.

Spirituality is *not Morality*.

People who don't dare be spiritual call themselves moral. Morality is the human criterion of character, spirituality is the divine. They may coincide—they oftener conflict. That is, morality does the conflicting—God can't conflict with anybody or anything. To obey the moral law may be more immoral than to transgress it—if we obey it, as most people do, under protest or external pressure. Electricity kills a good many people, but you don't blame the current. Spirituality nullifies a good many laws—when they get where they don't belong.

Spirituality is *not Paucity*.

To be "poor in spirit" is not necessarily to be poor in pocket-book or in human tendencies. *To be anywhere scant is to be somewhere soulless.* The pauper and the ascetic have for ages been taken as the types of spiritual men. Spiritual—or just lazy and anaemic? No pauper can be spiritual who did not *first* have wealth to relinquish; no ascetic who did not *first* have passion to sublimize. The Oriental doctrine of Renunciation is responsible for much pseudo-spirituality. *Renounce* and *relinquish* are two different words. The true mystic often relin-quishes, *never* renounces. No authentic Messiah ever renounced the world—he only relinquished it on visioning the Infinite. But his devotees, seeing the bare act and blind to the incentive, have renounced for the *mere sake of renouncing.* A very crude illustration here. Suppose two little brothers have a Noah's Ark between them, with a fine menagerie of wooden animals carefully painted and varnished. One little brother gets mad some day and smashes his collection of animals; *he renounces.* The other little brother is presented the same day with a live dog or pony; *he relinquishes.* You see it's all in the motive, don't you? Besides, the second little brother has left his wooden animals for some other little boy to play with for awhile—a little boy that hasn't any live dog or pony. So many little boys there are like that—little boys, and big boys—*and* little boys who call themselves big boys.

All these things Spirituality is not; what then is it?

Spirituality is a man's *permeability with the inflow and outflow of the Deific.* It is the capacity of an incarnate soul to do two things; first to isolate itself from sense-elements and become stored with the primal pulse of Omnipotence; then to infuse itself thus charged into whatever or whomever it touches. Not theological at all, you see—not necessarily human. Any being is spiritual whose *perceptions* are all open *heavenward* and whose *faculties* are equally open *earthward.* Brain and body must be still while soul receives its enduement; then must brain and body rouse every atom for the materializing of the message. A dormant faculty in the brain; a dead fibre in the body; a thought of failure in the mind; a feeling of constraint in the heart; a stoppage anywhere, however slight, will make a man less spiritual by so much. It is a *moral impossibility for a lazy man to be spiritual.* Perhaps this explains why so few clergymen are spiritual.

One point in particular would I dwell on.

It is this: *sense and soul are inseparable.*

Read the studies of Havelock Ellis in Sex; truths gleaned the world over by a man absolutely unprejudiced and strictly scientific. Learn how *religious exaltation* is but a finer form of *sex-transport.* The trances of adepts are attained through the sublimizing of sex-power. The visions of seers pass down the same way that visions of sex-imagination pass up. The rhapsodies of poets quiver with Truth the Eternal Feminine like as their bodies thrill with the touch of the Woman they love. Spirituality is surcharged with sex. And the sexless are invariably the soulless.

You quote the advice of great religious teachers who had renounced the delights of sense? Yes—but their *souls* never told them to. Only another case of *brain interfering* between soul and body. The *brain* of a man unduly *objectifies* the sex of a man; the *brain* of a woman unduly *subjectifies* the sex of a woman. Indeed all sensual excess inculpates the brain—not the body. Since it arises from the *mental habit* of coaxing sense instead of heeding soul.

Next to the human tongue, is the human brain the greatest mischief-maker on earth. We can't abolish it just at present—we need it in our business. But we've yet to learn to keep it in its place; with *soul overseeing* and *body working right alongside.*

"How to become spiritual?" has been the perennial problem of the church authorities.

And their usual answer? "By Fasting and Prayer."

Let me echo that answer, affirming it absolutely correct. Only they didn't know how to fast—nor how to pray. God gave them the idea, so it was good. But they asked men instead of

Nature to help them work it out; and that was bad. Here is a typical case. The Church of Scotland appointed July 23, 1835 as a "Day of Humiliation," to be observed as a General Fast Day everywhere. But they were *scared* into it—they'd been raising trouble with their neighbors and were getting the worst of the scuffle. So it appeared about time to purloin some of the panoply of God. They evidently thought God would be so tickled to see them starving themselves He would forget to watch the clerical vassals deputed to steal His armor. We observe this attitude of expectation in a certain famous sermon delivered apropos to the Day; the preacher recurring constantly to the "vengeance of Heaven" and the "forgiveness of sins." Also he declares they undertook the Fast from a "sense of duty" and to honor the "spirit of the forefathers." I hope the forefathers felt better after the Fast—the record forgot to say.

Now of course we don't believe in the "mortification and self-denial" theory, or its consequent sack-cloth-and-ashes practice. Yet the General Fast Day has its advantages—as those sects that still observe it will bear witness. *It obviates adverse suggestion*—nobody is constantly urging you to eat and prophesying starvation if you don't. It also ensures *physiological benefit in the guise of religious blessing.* Which will be needed so long as men depend on a blind faith, being ignorant equally of body and soul. Moreover it gives you *something better than your symptoms to think about.* A point overlooked by some of our professional Fasters. Never mind if your worship be superstition—a man-made God is better than a Devil-made man.

What is the "Conquest Fast?"

It is a *combination of the early Church Fast with the modern Therapeutic Fast.* It attempts to avoid the errors of each yet retain the benefits of both. However more or less it avails thus for you, the Conquest Fast has done this for me; it has *spiritualized Spirituality.* I never knew before what the word meant. I could accept neither the austerities of the church's theory nor the carnalities of the world's practice. I am now assured, through the visions of the Conquest Fast, that *the church must find its own body while the world must find its own soul.* Separated, neither the world nor the church can be truly spiritual. United, they may express Deity sublimely and inaugurate Heaven on earth.

A spiritual man is all of this—and a good deal more.
1. He is *natural.*
2. He is *original.*
3. He is *energetic.*
4. He is *magnetic.*
5. He is *enthusiastic.*
6. He is *forceful.*
7. He is *tender.*
8. He is *liberal.*
9. He is *worldly-wise.*
10. He is *self-contained.*
11. He is *loving.*
12. He is *womanly.*

I am *not yet worldly-wise enough to be spiritual.* That's why I'm leaving Naturism and going into business. When this deficiency is supplied, I shall take up the next that needs looking after. Perhaps in fifty or a hundred years I shall be somewhere near spiritual. Even if not—it's a comfort to know what the word means; and to be satisfied with nothing less than the genuine.

FASTING FOR INSTINCT

CHAPTER XI.

Most people know so little because they think so much.

They *study* science instead of *learning* from Omni-science.

The chief object of a college curriculum seems to be so to block the "threshold of consciousness" that the soul cannot pass in and out freely. Yet the sill itself is left unplaned and the door unhinged—I suppose they think the fact that we get what we don't need is offset by the more glaring fact that we need what we don't get.

The lessons that last longest are the ones that impress themselves silently, carrying with them no conscious memories. We remember best what we never need recall.

The only infallible memory is the memory of Instinct—the only infallible judgment is the judgment of Instinct. What we have *felt* we remember by instinct—merely what we have *thought* must we recollect by reason. And, as you may have gathered already, I am assured that feeling is a much finer, truer, purer, surer, higher mode of perception than thought. Life is measured least by what we have done, more by what we have thought, more yet by what we have loved, most of all by what we have *felt*. *Love feels*—and knows. *Law reasons*—and is forever doubting, quibbling, denying.

Go to some meeting where reason runs riot—say the Manhattan Liberal Club, of New York City. What do you hear? A jargon of profitless sound; a clashing of brains on edge; a pitting of wild hypothesis against savage denunciation; a fusillade of facts athwart a blank wall of doubt; a charge of mental musketry; a sight of bleeding *souls* and an echo of their moaning;—then out again into the night. But the gloom you have left is darker than the night—nor dawns yet the day in the distance.

What a contrast when you and your sweetheart meet at the spot of your first trysting-place! How the very path is hallowed that you trod together. How the tree where you leaned stands straighter. How the moss is softer for the memory of her touch.

How the brook sings more joyously since it filled the cup that you and she first shared;—you know that was the day you discovered your sweetheart must always take a sip before you drank. Since the dew of her lips would purify and sweeten the flow from Arcadia's crystal fount.

If we only loved enough, the vividness of Love's remembrance would halo all the world! Then should we see with the eye of the Creator.

The average human is a nondescript creature, combining the dim memory of an animal with the dimmer prophecy of a god. At present he is neither animal, man nor god. He has lost his animal-instinct, he has not attained his god-consciousness, he is just in the process of developing his man-reason. So we observe him bumping about into all sorts of obstacles—including his neighbors—with the deftness of a June-bug and the farsightedness of a bat. He doesn't know he's a hybrid. But that's what's the matter. And he won't be acquainted with himself till he succeeds in tracing his ancestral lines more accurately.

Most of us witness in our own person a life-long struggle between reason and instinct. But there should be no conflict—there *is none* between *my* instinct and *my* reason. Only between *my* instinct and the *world's* reason. And if I would but stop the world's mouth or my own ears long enough to hear myself, I should find how perfectly *my* instinct and *my* reason work together.

To put it succinctly; for the journey of Life, we may say that *Reason draws the map, makes the time-table, and runs the train;* while *Instinct points the direction, fixes the destination, sets the clock and prepares the lunch.* Now there are rival roads in the realm of Reason—scores of them. And the trouble with us is we are forever asking the ticket-agent where we want to go. He doesn't know—hasn't the least idea. But naturally he sells us a ticket to the end of his line—that's his business. Then we discover that wasn't the place after all. So we come back and make another foolish try.

Here is the rule for reconciling Reason and Instinct.

Ask Instinct what to do—ask Reason how to do it. That is, Reason may direct but not dictate, may suggest but not sanction. In any case, however, of *apparent* conflict, trust Instinct rather than Reason. Spirit speaks to soul through Instinct, soul speaks to body through Impulse, body answers and obeys through Action. Reason, on the other hand, is simply the cry of the world —a voice from without, estranged from both Impulse and Action.

Instinct is the register of pre-incarnate experience—Reason is the shuttle of current experiment. That is, what we get rationally in this life we get instinctively or intuitively in the next. Instinct therefore may be assumed as much finer than Reason as a resurrected soul is assumed finer than a mortal of clay.

Reason is higher than Instinct only in the sense of being *supplementary* to it. Instinct must be the foundation of a sane life, as in animals so in men; Reason but adds another story or two to your structure. In reality, the "lower animals" are far more exemplary than the human race. Animals are absolutely true to themselves, in so far as they know; whereas men wittingly misuse and blaspheme body, mind and soul. Perfect fidelity to self is a finer, deeper, subtler thing than the average man ever dreamed of. A little illustration—very homely, but very apt.

I was recently obliged, out of courtesy, to dine at a large table where a score of people ate together. There were four kinds of acid food for a single meal—cottage cheese, grape jelly, oranges and cherries. I *instinctively* took the cheese and the jelly, refusing the fresh fruits. Most of the guests refused not one of the acids. After dinner, I happened to recall the four varieties of acid, and to reflect that the two I combined *from desire alone* were the only two that should combine for *digestibility alone.* Which means I have come so close to my soul that I cannot mistake its faintest whisper; nor need I empanel the brain to interpret.

Impulses are the sinews of the soul. How can sinews strengthen without exercise? Many a beautiful soul has been palsied with fearing to act on its impulses. Fearing lest the world call it emotional, sentimental, or sinful. Instinct and feeling are as inseparable as soul and body. But we have dwelt in our *brains* so long as to forget the oneness of soul and body. Instinct therefore is condemned as bestial, and feeling is ridiculed as irrational. Purblind humans! Too sickly to be animals—and too sanctimonious to be gods!

A recent illustration of the obtuseness of mentality;—in connection with Oscar Wilde's book *"De Profundis."* Never have I heard so sincere a cry from a soul in the depths of anguished feeling. Yet his own publishers in announcing the book, laid stress on what they termed "the peculiarly artificial nature" of the author. Truly our friends are our worst enemies. There is some hope when our foes misunderstand us; but not when our friends do—for they think they know us. To the few that understand, I am more than undescribable. I Am Nameless. Just an All-embracing Consciousness wherein they rest and fall asleep.

Impulses grow best in Dreamland. And that's where children live. Aren't you sorry you moved away?

Do you enjoy your pile of wood or stone as once you did your air-castle? Are you altogether at home—within four walls and a roof? Is there no part of you that mounts beyond the cupola, fleeing earth-constraint?

Most of the troubles that haunt men are ghosts of truths lost from childhood.

The purpose of our teaching children is that they may teach us without our knowing it. It is the mother who will not learn of her child that punishes him—for her own delinquency.

The crucial test of wisdom is the renunciation of knowledge. Not even a sage can stand this test—it takes a seer. No wonder a poor little mother is heavily weighed with foolish fears, superfluous advice, deadly warnings, and dismal precedents;—when the wisest of men dare not trust their own souls. And the babe has to suffer. How many things a child instinctively rebels at—things the mother *thinks* she knows but the child *knows* she doesn't know. Forced feeding; close confinement; bed-pins; safety-pins and responsibility-pins; bitter medicine; scratchy flannels; shoes and stockings; tight underwear and stiff outerwear; book-learning; church attendance; perfunctory prayer; social distinctions; hereditary vocation; regular duties; mute obedience; catering to authority; any sort of ology or ism; in short the fetters, the blinders, the threateners of the race, all of which take shape when we know too much and feel too little.

How anomalous to call a man a "grown-up"—him but a remnant of the largeness of childhood. The time will come when education will run like this:—INSTINCT FIRST, INSPIRATION SECOND, *Instruction third.* Since the body is most vital, soul next, brain least.

Let me quote right here extracts from a recent utterance of Professor Edgar L. Larkin, whose reputation as a pure scientist can but echo my consciousness as a pure mystic. "Three-fourths of the entire literature of the world is now obsolete. The discoveries being made hourly must have world-wide effect soon. Many of our habits and customs must be greatly modified, and others wiped out. The future school will be so unlike those we now have that one can scarcely realize the transformation. The sensitive mind of a poet can be ruined by three or four years of forced drill in geometry and analytics. And no teacher will be allowed, under heavy penalty, to attempt to teach any child or youth until its mind is examined by expert mentalists."

All of which tends toward the position outlined in this book.

To be called childlike is the greatest compliment payable to any man. It means he is simple, natural, sincere, spontaneous, cheerful, charitable, sympathetic, trustful, loving, idealistic. *And* instinctive.

Therefore is the promise of childlikeness by no means the least conferment tendered by the Conquest Fast.

Let me cite a few details.

1. *The Conquest Fast severs false relationships.* Either the thralldom of things or the pinch of personality prevents our living

naturally. But how can we see the yoke we bear while still we bear it? There are just two ways to treat an uncongenial atmosphere; change it or leave it. To change it means usually to match one against the multitude—a terrific strain and useless waste of energy. By lifting us bodily from our environ of doubt and hesitancy, the Conquest Fast puts us where we can create our own atmosphere by the natural outworkings of instinct.

2. *The Conquest Fast reveals the insignificance of the brain.* And this we must sense very strongly before we dare trust to our souls. We might liken the brain to a telegraphic instrument, and the soul to a Marconi transmitter. One needs a network of mental machinery—the other a single flash of sunlight. We shall probably never be able to dispense wholly with telegraph instruments. But nothing save the wireless can reach the ships at sea.

Many a barque that has set sail on the sea of Truth drifts today void of destination. Reach it with your brain you cannot— illumine it with your soul you may.

Before you light a lamp, you turn the wick low. Before God lights a soul is the soul prepared for the dim glow of instinct. A turn higher, as the flame brightens, and we have intuition. The next is inspiration. And at last, with the full brilliance of the soul's luminosity, shines the splendid beacon of revelation.

3. *The Conquest Fast refines the reasoning faculties.* A mystic needs reason as much as a materialist needs soul. And the Naturist often needs both. To attune your perceptions without developing your faculties is to put a gag between your lips and then ask you to read to us. It is *not* natural for a *human* being to live forever in the backwoods. He must mingle with men, must feel the spur of business activity, must whet his wits on financial problems, must learn to decide quickly, act firmly, and plan persistently.

Feeling must be *furthered* by thought. Deep emotional natures are often repressed, or expressed wrongly, through lack of reasoning power. Adolph Just, for instance, in his wonderfully helpful book *"Return to Nature,"* loses through *lack of logic* much of the ground gained through the leading of instinct. His message is true in the main—but often it fails to convince, because it is not cogent.

Now the Conquest Fast by the same process of clarification first frees the soul, then quickens the brain to fulfil the soul's behest. It should raise you to the acme of *all* your powers—or at least show you how to get there.

4. *The Conquest Fast perpetuates the joy of living.* I'm getting tired of being solemn—there's been a smile asking to come out for ever so long. When I go to "Advanced Thought" meetings—or used to, I know better now—I would feel myself freezing stiff from outside in. It's just as cold in the clouds as in the cellar. And when you *have* to be loving, you can't philosophize very long at a time.

If we aren't happy, we aren't whole. And to have the secret of wholeness is to have the secret of happiness. Whenever a doubt crosses my vision, or a chill threatens my heart, or the slightest discomfort irritates my body, I know at once where the stress of externals has closed in on my soul. I have repressed natural instinct and yielded before unnatural intellect; I have let the braggadocio of brute mentality parry the thrill of gentle Deity; I have somehow been less than myself. To regain my diminished stature and exult again in my suspended happiness, I have but to loosen the cumbrance with a mighty pulse of truer purpose. Then the next time be utterly myself. Whence this soul-certainty? From the Conquest Fast.

The bird was born to sing and to soar. Just this the bird does —and is happy.

The flower was born to be sweet and be beautiful. Just this the flower is—and has happiness to share.

What I was born to do and to be, only that in its fulness suffices. Always happy I if I measure up to myself.

Let us smile.

FASTING FOR INSPIRATION

CHAPTER XII.

God remembers Man when Man forgets the world.

Which is but a briefer way of saying that when Self has been ascended into, all that is not Self falls behind. For *the inspirational life is the natural life,* and our souls suffocate in any other.

Men who call themselves "sensible"—how strange, since they possess least sensibility—may doubt or deny Inspiration. But still their souls suffocate—you can see it in their eyes.

While many a man who disputes any premise of the "supernatural," himself works under inspiration. At rare intervals Love does manage to shine through the thick black shutter of Logic—perhaps a flower, a strain of music, a baby's voice, or a woman's kiss has found a way past the lattice.

By inspiration I do not mean irrationality.

Most people make the two identical. Therefore do they dread the vaguest hint of seizure by the Subliminal. They dread because they do not understand. Which is tautology in the extreme; since the one object of human dread is that gruesome shroud of Ignorance.

By inspiration I may mean irresponsibility.

People deplore this also—from equal lack of understanding. But as this appears harmless to them, the voices of God that come to its possessor they graciously stifle under the mantle of charity, while whispering that open-sesame to pity—"He's irresponsible." There are compensations however—your friends leave you severely alone. They would call it "severely"—you call it mercifully. When people can't pin to you, they can't stick you.

Inspiration is supposed to accompany religious frenzy, hence conduce to insanity. Religious frenzy however is the *inability to use* Inspiration rather than the capacity to receive it. It's the whirring of the engine when a cog has slipped, and the power spends itself in vain.

Half-hearted or hypocritical lovers make public protestations of affection; real lovers let silence speak for them—silence and service.

So here. God does not authenticate monomaniacs.

And yet; I have had a howling dervish, with his outlandish dance, give me more genuine soul-thrills than a polished theologian ever felt all his life. Inspiration goes when Education comes. I mean of course orthodox education—anything "orthodox" being mostly spurious.

I affirm without hesitation that the naked savage in his ignorant state lives a more inspired life than the average churchmember.

Inspiration is commonly confused with occultism or creedism. A psychic thinks herself inspired because she is gifted with powers not yet explained by science. She errs wofully. The truly inspired soul never calls itself "clairvoyant" or "clairaudient." The possession of such faculties puts one in touch, not with the Infinite, but only with higher entities on the mortal plane. To be extremely psychic is to be extremely uninspired and uninspiring. It takes more than telepathy to hold commune with God.

Neither is Inspiration confined to creed. It is often limited by creed—as in most of the cases the Bible records. You believe, for instance, in a personal Deity; you'll get no universal truth. Even Infinite Light cannot penetrate a stone wall. Its area is enclosed by the bounds of your soul-window, its splendor can but mark the clearness of your mind-glass.

This fact is generally forgotten by those who have outgrown churches. Freed perhaps from the prison walls and windows of race-belief, they have blindly plunged into the *gloomier maze of their own mentality*. Where there is no belief at all. Better to catch an occasional gleam through a window thick with grime than to grope forlorn in outer darkness.

Inspiration is usually saturated with superstition. Artists, poets, prophets, priests have claimed to be inspired by special dispensation. And when common mortals presumed to question such a superhuman being, he has promptly and eloquently invoked the wrath of the Almighty to protect the chosen one from assaults of the unclean. On the one hand, this travesty.

On the other, equal excess of modesty. Many an everyday human, that works with the hands for the daily bread, is daily inspired. The world probably calls such a one "emotional, childish, simple-minded." Because, as I have already said, the world does not understand.

Inspiration, moreover, seldom works itself out *through the same soul that received it.* This because of the soul's lack of symmetry, splendid body and superb brain being required to *give* inspiration no less than receptive spirit to *get* it. Most of the world's seers have been physically inert. Their besetting sin has been to contemplate their souls. Not a common sin, to be sure; but a poignant one wherever found. Whoever indulges it can be but partially inspired.

Since I have attained the Cosmic Consciousness I have often been tempted to retire finally from human activity. There is so little on earth to hold me it seems a waste of time to stay.

Then I make straight for Lower Broadway. And it doesn't take long for the man's ambition to rise, supplementing the god's aspiration, thus leaving me an all-round human.

Not the presence of Poesy makes a bard unbalanced—*but the absence of Philosophy.* Don't blame Poesy—blame Philosophy that it hasn't got around yet.

In this connection, let me tell you something. Put your ear very close—it's a secret between me and you. "To a real poet, the average business man or society woman looks even more unbalanced than a mystic looks to dowager or financier." Moreover, I've sort of a dim idea that God would agree with the mystic. Not every mystic, understand. Some of them have malaria, and don't know the difference.

Let us dwell a moment longer on this point of asymmetry.

To be conscious of soul is to be unconscious of both body and brain. Which controverts the claims of both Physical Culturist and Advanced Psychologist.

But to *remain* unconscious of brain and body, one must first have been conscious in every atom of both—*fully, actively, regnantly* conscious.

Spirit moves most when form moves least. But form must commence to move immediately Spirit ceases. And unless form has already learned how—the behest of Spirit fails of accomplishment.

This is too abstruse—let's see if an illustration won't make it clearer. Take the flash of lightning that momentarily relieves a midnight storm. If it comes often enough, you can find your way home by it. How? First wait for the light—then follow as far as you can see. But to be guided aright, *you must move* while the flash is yet upon you. How far would it help you if you hadn't learned to walk? Or if you stopped because the path looked steep and slippery?

Inspiration is most often nullified right here.

The soul that has the beautiful vision lacks the courage or capability to carry it out. The soul that hasn't it therefore doubts its existence. Some more practical mortal shall materialize the ideal of the visionary—since no ideal is ever lost. But by that time it has ceased to be direct inspiration. So the world cannot trace it. Only the dreamer *knows a dream's dynamics.*

In short, expression must succeed impression, power must re-enforce perception, activity must lend poise and assurance to sensitivity. Not otherwise can the illumined soul be true to its vision. Not otherwise can the unillumined soul be led to seek the Light.

With this very brief and incomplete preface, let us now consider the Conquest Fast.

I cannot guarantee that the Fast will conduct you to the Fount of Inspiration—Omniscience has a way of avoiding specified routes and choosing Its Own. Inspiration passes down as many avenues as individuals pass up. For a survey of the various means of access to the Subliminal, I suggest very earnestly a study of the Vedânta Philosophy. It lacks heart; it hampers itself with nomenclature; it fails to develop the individual. Nonetheless, Vedânta is the broadest and best system of scientific faith yet formulated; for such as are still subject to system.

I am entirely convinced however that an *indeterminate* Fast is the one and only sure medium for utter absorption in the Universal. You must not only stop eating—you must absolutely forget food. Forget everything and everybody else of course; I emphasize food because we are in deepest bondage to it. The thing most dear is the thing most dangerous.

You may have a thing until you must. *Then you mustn't.*

But there is always recompense. The gods let many a man remain poor that they themselves may sustain him. This is the psychology of that proverbially pitiful "crust in a garret." If geniuses always knew why, when and how to forego their cake, Providence would never restrict them to a crust. But geniuses are peculiarly fond of cake—for some of them it has to be extra sugared and spiced. Then nurse Nature prescribes bread and water. Good for the genius, perhaps good for posterity. Hard though, very hard on the genius's near neighbors.

The spiritual and the sensuous are so subtly interblended that few souls can distinguish earth-appeal from heaven-appeal. Fewer still can respond to one without renouncing the other. The finest lesson of life is to adjust the balance between soul and sense.

In general this maxim is effective; *to make soul less elusive, make body less obtrusive.* If anything can reduce both brain and body to their proper place, it is assuredly the Conquest Fast. Not self-control, self-denial, self-subordination; rather self-equation, self-expression, self-exaltation.

In reading this book, some folks will say I have drawn largely on my imagination to picture what the Conquest Fast will do.

I want to nail that fallacy right here.

And I have the spikes to do it with.

Among many services the Fast rendered me, let me mention three of the most vital.

1. *It marked a complete change in my prose style.*

Three years ago I was mournful in my writings. I was pessimistic. I was didactic. I was rhetorical. I was attenuated—in phraseology as in physiognomy. It took me a dozen sallies in verbosity before I'd beat about the bush long enough to reach the point. Then it wasn't the one I wanted. And Heaven knows nobody else wanted it.

Shortly after the Fast, I noticed that punctuation points began to get less scarce. Now and then, too, a smile would creep in. Very shyly at first, a little uncertain about feeling at home. Lately the smiles have grown so bold they actually flirt with me. More wonderful still, I pat them on the check, tell them how pretty they look, and not to hurry away. Really smiles aren't dangerous when you know how to treat them. They resemble women in that respect.

2. *The Fast developed my poetic gifts.*

Prior to the summer when I fasted, I had never written a single poem. The nearest to it being that concatenation of frightful utterances termed "college yell."

In the ten months immediately following the Fast, *over two hundred poems* were transcribed. Twenty-seven came in a single week, eight in a single day. This unparalleled volume of verse I attribute directly to the Thirty-Day Fast.

Don't conclude that Fasting will make everybody a poet. At least let us hope not—so long as barbers and magazine editors have to make a living.

But whatever your special talents may be, these should be revealed through the Fast. It may be remarked in passing that if you do happen to be a poet, then a successful experience in Fasting may prove other than ornamental. It's so much easier to do without things when you want to than when you have to.

3. *The Fast disclosed my life-work.*

The one lesson that stuck to me while in college was that I should likely go to the poor-house when I got out.

This lesson isn't in the curriculum, being reserved for the first year in the world's post-graduate school. But I was precocious and got mine as a Freshman. It lodged to stay too—not even a fraternity initiation could blot it out altogether. If I wished to dishearten the most incorrigible optimist, I should propose this test:—"Let us hope for the day when colleges teach a man to be of some use, to the world or himself."

The only thing unique about a successful man is that he has found his place. Most misfits are made so by their education or surroundings—if left to themselves they would gravitate to their work. Here again *brain conflicts with soul.* And soul is left wounded and weeping for a lifetime. Regret is mostly inspiration denied till its opportunity passed; if only we could realize this on the eve of denial instead of the day after.

But to come to the point;—is it possible I am still addicted to circumlocution?

The Conquest Fast revealed to me; first, my oneness with Omnipotence; second, my work in the world; third, my best and quickest means of identifying the two. Ever since the Fast, the goal has grown clearer, and the avenues to it broader. At no single time have there been less than six possibilities awaiting me; any one of which would have led ultimately to the object of desire. Compare this with the average man's anxiety in "getting a job," his trepidation in holding it, his despair at losing it. *I own* any "job" I want anywhere. But I don't want it—unless through it I may serve the ends of Truth. Then it comes to me— I need never beg for it.

To be inspired is to know myself and be myself. Any soul thus inspired commands whatever situation it chooses. Since all the world is waiting for it.

———

To-day, as I write this chapter, I am beginning another Fast. I may eat again next week—perhaps not till the week after—certainly not while the cry of my soul for Truth can still the call of my body for food.

My brain is clouded, my body irritated; these conditions usually marking the first days of a Fast.

But my heart is light, my soul radiantly happy. Already angels' voices woo me from a distance. Symphonies no ear can sense, visions no eye can bear, eternities of glory no mortal can attain; a rapturous blending with the Spirit Source of worlds and stars and solar systems; is not this worth more than a morsel of food on the tip of the tongue?

FASTING FOR LOVE

CHAPTER XIII.

Love is the supreme and ultimate Mystery of the Universe.

Nothing in this world is so little understood or so much misunderstood.

Of all things most beautiful yet terrible, powerful yet fragile, beneficent yet selfish, tender yet savage, tranquil yet tumultuous, eloquent yet mute, brave yet fearful, eternal yet fickle, sincere yet evasive, ideal yet practical, universal yet personal, reverent yet intimate, divine yet human.

Understand Love—and you have solved the riddle of existence.

Exalt Love—and you have reached the very heart of religion.

Welcome Love—and you have opened your arms to the angels.

Live Love—and you have won the hearts of men.

Deserve Love—and you have felt the caress of the Infinite Comforter.

Embody Love—and you have known the utmost joy of the Creator of worlds.

Trust Love—and you have placed your life in the keeping of Omniscience.

All the woes of this world arise from either the repression or the perversion of Love. About three-fourths from too little of the right kind, and one-fourth from too much of the wrong kind. The so-called virtuous apportion the three-fourths, the so-called vicious the one-fourth. And it's a question which element is more effective as a woe-producer.

A pauper is a man who doesn't love his work, not having found it.

A criminal is a man who doesn't love his finest ideal, having allowed some grosser to usurp its place.

A reformer is a man who doesn't love Humanity.

A lawyer is a man who doesn't love Justice.

A doctor is a man who doesn't love Nature.

A theologian is a man who doesn't love God.

You observe I put the reformers, lawyers, doctors and theologians in the same category with the pauper and the criminal. I think they belong about half-way between. They are not so poor as the pauper, nor so honest as the criminal. They none of them know the joy of living. You won't love to live until you live to love.

Now the reason Love is so generally misunderstood and misapplied is because Love is limitless while every lover is circumscribed by limitations. And we unconsciously confuse our judgment of Love with our opinion of the lover. We can feel, recognize and answer only so much of Love as we ourselves have experienced. Which is oh so little with most of us. We are like children trying to guess the ocean-depths by the amount of spray that moistens the shore where we build our sand-houses.

I ask no surer judgment of a man than his own judgment of Love. Or a woman either. Because the average woman is as hard, as narrow, as unresponsive as the average man is gross, and clumsy, and disenchanting. The man is mute of soul, the woman of brain and body. Each is a cripple. You can't love either without a shudder. A shudder for you and a tremor for them. The pity of it is that in the depths of every human soul rises feebly an unutterable longing to love and be loved. So that he who fears, degrades or scorns Love fears, degrades or scorns himself. No wonder he is uncomfortable—letting his brain crowd his soul into some dark, unwholesome recess of his being. As a matter of fact, those who ridicule lovers are but trying to hide their envy of lovers. And if you watch closely, you can always see the smile of scorn droop at the corners—as if weeping for the kiss that never came.

Some one asks: "What is Love?"

But there is no answer—*for such as need ask.* Love's only interpreters are Love's exemplars. And to these, words are not necessary. You can feel Love, you can sense Love, you can look

Love, you can smile Love, you can touch Love, you can breathe Love, you can live Love;—but you can never tell Love.

Love is God. And God is undefinable.

Men have printed, cut and pasted thousands of labels to designate God. But whenever they thought to affix one, God wasn't there. So they had to take whatever was handy that looked most like God.

It's the same way with Love. Indeed a religious denomination is a device for measuring how far men have shut Love out of their lives. Did you ever hear of a Protestant rose, a Jewish canary, or a Catholic sunbeam? No more can you call sectarian any *human* life whose soul is sweet, whose message clear, whose heart radiant. Such a being of effluence you can never limit, never define, never regulate, never standardize, never reduce to tangible terms. All the world is too small to contain the love of a Godlike soul. Think you to constrict the flow of a mountain freshet in Springtime by a few legal, conventional or moral timbers built into the bank. When the surge comes from Up Yonder, snap go the barriers, dyke, dam and all; while the land is whelmed in a turbulent sea of billowy might.

How many geniuses have loved this way! To be pitifully misunderstood and cruelly condemned. Great elemental natures, filled with a mother-longing too big to be cramped by custom or cowed by opinion, how gloriously they have loved. And how fiendishly been throttled.

If the few splendid souls that dare love always knew how, the many scant souls that do not dare would awaken to their need. But mistakes are so often confused with motives. And we fear to trust the motives lest we repeat the mistakes.

Love is infinitely more than any one human's conception of Love. And we must fix this fact in mind before assuming to discuss Love.

Love is more than affection. Affection calls for some specific object of endearment, and vanishes with the object; Love lavishes itself impartially on the whole world. Affection is personal, changeable, transient; Love is universal, steadfast, eternal. Affection asks to be cherished quite as much as to cherish; *Love asks nothing but the privilege of loving.* Affection twines itself most closely about human relationships; Love finds its fullest fruition beyond the human race.

Love is more than sympathy. Sympathy deplores, pities, or commiserates. Love understands. And understanding never does any of these things. Love feels more than any mortal can feel— more of rapture, more of anguish. But Love is silent through it all. For Love knows that *just to be understood* is the finest, sweetest, rarest kind of sympathy treasured by the human soul. You may suffer with the sufferer—but only that he may in turn rejoice with you. And if you have not learned to smile while suffering—better steel yourself and not suffer.

Love is more than service. How many a harried housewife and irritable mother needs to learn this lesson. To minister to the body is often to stultify the soul. Rents in the heart are more costly than rents in a garment. And physical ease may be secured at the price of spiritual unrest. To inspire our fellows to trust, help and develop themselves—this is a higher service than running errands or prosecuting the weekly sweep. Many an anxious Martha waits in vain for the reward of her material forethought, while some sweet-faced Mary receives the blessing that follows only the outpouring of the heart.

Love is more than loyalty. Love is the one expansive force irresistible. So that of all created beings, lovers must grow. And if they cannot grow together, they must grow apart. Loyalty is the exalting of person above principle; Love is the overshadowing of person by principle. A kind of incomplete loving may hold together a very young soul and a very old soul unawakened. But when the awakening comes, they will separate as night from day. The young soul will probably possess mental acumen—for only young souls glory in that sort of thing. And the old soul will probably be simple, natural, childlike—for only old souls are wise enough to be themselves. The world therefore, being very young indeed, will laud the blind loyalty of the infant soul, while disparaging the far-sighted sincerity of the experienced soul.

In the five years I have been unfolding, I have entered and outgrown that many circles of friends. The few friends I have now I was not ready for then; the many friends I had then are not ready for me now. And so we part—I, at least, with a smile and a Godspeed. The mission of friendship is to teach us how dearly we may cherish something without wanting to own it. How many of us are learning that we cannot, must not own our friends? It is easy to smile when Love comes—easy and beautiful. But when Love goes—never from the soul, only from the brain or the body—then it is not so easy. Yet more beautiful. The Love that lets is the rarest and most precious. Nor is this sacrifice. Love is Love that *asks* neither recognition nor return— but that *gets* both. We can never really lose what or whom we have really loved.

Love is more than passion. Love between sweethearts cannot live without passion. This every woman needs to feel. But Love between sweethearts cannot live on passion alone. And this every man needs to feel. Passion born in the soul is divine. Passion born in the brain or the body is abortive—humanly abortive. Nature says "Be utterly passionate—but be pure first." Humanity says "You should not be passionate. For if you are, you cannot be pure."

It is perhaps true that women are not passionate because men are not pure. It is no less true that *men are not pure because women are not passionate.* To be natural is to be both. Men force Love—and are impure. Women repress Love—and are impure. There is no choice.

And yet, being a man, I cannot help seeing more vividly the grossness of men's mistakes in the relation of soul to sex. How few men can send their souls through the thrill of their touch! How many women long for lovers who can. No man ever realizes that tenderness is power till he learns how to caress his sweetheart.

The reason men's bodies fail to attract women is that men's bodies fail to express men's souls. And your sweetheart must have your soul first. You satisfy the soul of a woman—and all of her is yours. Neglect or insult her soul—and none of her is yours. You complain she is cold, artificial, uninteresting? No, not that. You are coarse. You are stupid. You are unfeeling. You are too much man. And not enough baby, not enough woman, not enough god.

I believe in the absolute abandon of Love. But I also believe that *reverence without freedom is less of an evil than freedom without reverence.* Freedom is always a possibility to be achieved; while reverence, once lost, can never be recovered. A "Freelover" is a person so heterogeneous he hasn't any other half. So he goes about searching for an assortment of fractions wherewith to complete his own deficiencies. Every pure woman should shrink from him as from a viper.

Truth lies half-way between the ascetic and the Freelover.

He who frowns at sex never felt its ecstacy; he who jests at sex never felt its sanctity. Sex cannot be enjoyed and used to the full *until you have sublimized it to the fineness of the rapture of religion.* Such a wedding needs no trousseau or bridal party. The Recording Angel issues no marriage certificates. Betrothals in Heaven are authorized by Instinct, sanctified by Love, consummated by Abandon, and witnessed by Silence. Such a ceremony is lawless, wordless, thoughtless.

But before a marriage can be made in Heaven, both the lovers must have lived there long enough to become naturalized. This makes the cases so rare we really don't need to consider them. Besides, mere earth-dwellers wouldn't understand them anyway.

Love is more than wisdom. Only those wise enough to be loving are loving enough to be wise. The wisest people in this world are children, poets, idealists, and virgin mothers. Their wisdom isn't the college kind to be sure—it's the kind God gave them. You never found God studying at college or compiling facts from a library. God's enlightenment shines straight through the heart and soul; it hasn't time to filter through that miasmic mass of judicial jelly we call a brain.

Love and light begin with the same letter. And end with the same thrill. Your complexion will be whiter if you always stay in a darkened room. But the child of Nature risks even a little sunburn in order to be out-of-doors. Wisdom counselled Love—"See these scars and be cautious." Love replied—"You show the scars—and regret them? You never loved!"

Love may wound. But Love always leaves a soothing balm that makes you feel better than before the hurt. The dearest memento in my possession is a little scar once impressed on my flesh by Some One I love.

Love though is not all transcendental or sentimental. Love is pre-eminently practical. It does things. Being Infinite Energy, it must. *Every great success is but the growth of a great love.* Love for an individual, or for an ideal, or for the Infinite. And the size of your success always measures the size of the thing you love. Love your family—and your success will be to supply its wants. Love your country—and your success will be to administer public office. Love your race—and your success will be to immortalize your name in business, art or invention. Love your Spirit Source—and your success will be to incarnate Its splendor for the emulation of mankind.

Human knowledge may instruct. Human prestige may support. But Love alone both illumines and empowers. And the origin of Love is superhuman—whether you like the word or not.

———

Having taken this bare glimpse of the province of Love, let us inquire how its expression is enhanced by means of the Conquest Fast.

1. *The Conquest Fast restores the solar plexus to its natural state.* A human can't love normally with an abnormal solar plexus, this being the emotional brain. Now you won't find a perfect solar plexus save in about two individuals; a little child

uncivilized by wrong clothing, food and thought, and a man just completing a protracted Fast. Everybody else is stuffed inside and choked outside. And the delicate nerve-centre you need to love with is disabled, poisoned, benumbed.

You may have tried to "wake the solar plexus" by breathing exercises, "affirmations," and so forth. Good. All good. But you'll have to heal that dilated stomach, reduce that enlarged liver, quiet that inflamed digestive tract, before your affection-dynamo can put itself in working order.

The very process of digestion is quickened by the act of loving. It is the soul that assimilates food—not the body. And *the more you love, the less food does the soul need* to retain its mortal habiliment. Thus a wee lunch of bread, cheese and kisses is physiologically more wholesome, more strengthening, more satisfying than any table-d'hôte dinner in a table-d'hôte atmosphere. Particularly if you and your sweetheart prepare the little meal together, then eat it in an upper room of a cottage built on a mountain-peak, or facing the placid stretch of the sea.

Indeed the only time a self-conscious soul cares not to eat alone is when his really truly sweetheart is by his side. She is not company—she is his own heart and flesh.

2. *The Conquest Fast eliminates alien elements.* Love finds two chief hindrances to its natural expression; *food-poison* in the body and *fact-poison* in the brain. We swallow what custom feeds us, we believe what superstition tells us. As a result we are either *too pale to love passionately*—as on a woman's diet of tea and charlotte russe; or *too dense to love purely*—as on a man's diet of sirloin and French fry; or at least too confused to love spontaneously—as on anybody's diet either of romantic or of "scientific" literature, both being misleading.

Nothing but a long Fast will clear out all this rubbish, and enable a human to love like the god-animal that a human is. It clarifies both brain and body. In so doing, it liberates the soul for fresh activity.

3. *The Conquest Fast brightens the individual aura and certifies the individual vibration.* So-called "mismating" in marriage is but the constant attrition of undeveloped or insincere individuals. The soul that has found itself rings true. The soul that answers the vibration must also ring true. When these two mate, we have an affinity—a marriage made in Heaven, whether on earth or not.

In short, if your soul is a blue, a white, or a yellow, yet too weak and dim to be itself, you may take on the muddy brown of the personalities about you. Then when you come to love, you and the brown will be hopelessly mixed. And while you are working out the darker tinge that is really not you, your sweetheart will become disenchanted.

Now an extreme Fast separates you from all that is not you. It puts you on a new basis with the world. It does in reality what the orthodox churchman claims "conversion" will do. It alienates you from unreal friendship, and attracts to you the genuine. It identifies the desires of your heart with the dictates of your "conscience"—whatever and wherever that hypothesis may be. It makes Love synonymous with life. Because the fuller the life, the fuller the love.

4. *The Conquest Fast invests the real with the ideal.* No chasm in life is so hard to bridge as Love's hiatus between the ideal and the real. We love the ideal symbolized in a friend, but we think we love the mere personality. Then when the human side disappoints, we lose faith in the divine. I think there is nothing sadder than to see the capacity for belief in a lovely woman crushed to atoms because the trust in her girlish ideal has been shattered. An ideal is only a trellis whereon our affections may flower. To serve its purpose it *must* be outgrown. Should our love-nature be less aspiring than that of the morning-glory?

Now a mystic is never cast down by the destruction or desertion of the tangible. The breath of his life is the inspiration of the Unseen. The Conquest Fast should make you at least somewhat of a mystic. Enough so as to prevent your substituting the real for the ideal, or ever expecting ultimate satisfaction from sense-delights. You cannot divorce ideal from real, any more than you can cleave sun from shadow. But you can learn this: that while *comfort* seeks the shade, *growth* demands the sunlight. Yet in Love, as in Nature, the shade cannot lessen a flower's chlorophyll. Nor the sun bestow those dewy sweets of dawn or twilight. Love's repose forever alternates with Love's fever. Thus also the leaning on the real with the straining toward the ideal.

5. *The Conquest Fast equates personal and universal.* To be able to love Some One, love with all your heart, mind, soul and body—then to say good-bye if need be at the foot of the mountain, and go up alone to meet God; this is the ideal.

The all-round lover forgets the world in loving his sweetheart; then forgets his sweetheart in loving the world; then forgets both in loving the Infinite.

She may call him unreasonable in the third forgetting. She will surely call him cruel in the second. But he mustn't mind— if she weren't limited some way, she wouldn't do for his sweetheart.

Nothing teaches non-attachment so vividly as the Conquest Fast. It reveals the twin-necessity of utter absorption and utter separation. *All man one moment, all god the next;* this is the pendulum through which symmetry swings. The pious folk won't understand the first extreme, nor the worldly folk the second. But symmetry is never understood.

To be understood is to be defined. To be defined is to be limited. I am Limitless.

6. *The Conquest Fast expands the love-nature.* I always loved the hills, the sea, and the stars. Loved them more than I loved mortals. But before my long Fast, the hills came first, the sea next, and the stars last.

The order is reversed now. My love has largely outgrown the earthly ambition of the hills, and has merged into the heavenly calm of the eternal altitudes.

That is not all. Every tiny thing that grows has become my next of kin. The animals of the forest are more my friends than the humans of the city. I do not need the companionship of men. Indeed, only he understands fellowship who is never lonely when alone. I am my own inspiration—if you but let me be myself.

It is the lesser loves that fail to satisfy. And the sooner we express the largest love of which we are capable, the sooner will we realize health, happiness and *the dauntlessness of sincerity.*

7. *The Conquest Fast reveals the divinity of Love.* I used to be very intolerant toward the sinner. But I had not suffered enough, then. We never do understand the sinner until we ourselves have felt we must love, yet do not know what or how. Then we discover what salvation means—not a moral repentance, but a physical and mental regeneration.

He who loves wrongly because he must love is more Godlike than he who appears righteous because he cannot love. And when, through this long Fast, you have come close enough to the Heart of God, you will feel how every Love-impulse that animates us thrilled first from that Infinite Heart. Henceforth there is just one work for you—to reveal men to themselves, that they may love always and utterly as their souls impel. No stoppage in brain or body, no restraint from outside, no error from ignorance, no hesitation from fear.

Only Love, pure, powerful and perfect, as it shines in the sun, blossoms in the flower, laughs in the brook, sings in the bird, dreams in the star, soothes in the silence, and beckons in the blush immortal of a loving woman's cheek.

*TWENTY RULES FOR SANE FASTING

Rule 1—*Don't.*

Spell it out so as to remember it better; D-O-N- apostrophe T, *Don't.*

What? Thirteen long chapters commending the Fast with an unction unequalled—then one little word upsetting it all? Final proof, surely, that the author is unbalanced as well as unbridled.

Thank you, thank you. Some more, please. I'm getting so used to misjudgments that they taste kind of good—like olives after you've stroked away the preliminary pucker. Understand I don't consider olives wholesome. Yet they might keep one from starving.

If I wanted to be mean, I could get back at you for calling me crazy. I could say that these Rules referred to *Sane* Fasting, and that the prohibition merely implied doubt as to your eligibility. But I'll be generous and not even hint it—although it were true.

Seriously, there is reason in this hortatory paradox. Because in all probability you will have been unduly influenced by my interpretation of the Fast, and not sufficiently dominated by your own attitude toward it. Let us speak very frankly. During the past six years I have met in one way or another thousands of human beings that called themselves "advanced"—in Nature Cure, Physical Culture, New Thought, Oriental Philosophy, Divine Science or elsewise. Out of that number I know *less than a score* whom I deem *ready for the Conquest Fast.* Insofar of course as any short-sighted mortal can judge for another. No devotee, defender, or apostle is ever quite balanced. Enthusiasm

---

* I don't believe in Rules. That's why it's safe to give them. Safe for you—I find it dangerous for me to feel safe. But Rules are necessary for machine-made men. Until, therefore, you have disconnected your component parts from their custom-made mould and assembled them after your own plan: you will need Rules. This is only a harmless Rhetorical You—not a poisonous personal you.

has to run in a rut. But unless you have *enough ruts* to turn it in, you're sure to wear the one so deep you can't see out.

Do you believe in being all god, *or* all man, *or* all animal, as the impulse moves? And do you know how to be? Do you dare to be? Then, and then only, are you prepared to appreciate and experience *Sane* Fasting. When brain, heart, body and soul each knows its place and is wise enough to keep to it. If, irrespective of anything I have said, your own Higher Self tells you to take the extreme Fast, then do it. And triumph everlastingly. But never suffer your lesser self to be persuaded by any species of plausible diction or vicarious enthusiasm.

We might apply the simile of a relay journey to the destination reached by the Conquest Fast. There are three stations, *Self-Healing, Self-Empowering, Self-Illumining.* With the boulevard of Self-Enjoying connecting them. The first station, *Self-Healing,* is but a little way off. You can reach it by various means. You may don the sweater of Physical Culture—and sprint for it. You may hire the hose-cart of Hydropathy—and joggle to it. You may mount the fleshless old gray mule of Osteopathy— and creep toward it. You may recline on the stuffed stretcher of Christian Science—and be carried thither. Any way to get there. All depends on how you're built, what's the matter with you— *and* how much you'll spend on drayage. All these vehicles will get you there—sometime. Then *leave you there*—every time. Can't any of them take you to the second station, *Self-Empowering.* And the third stage, *Self-Illumining,* is out of their reckoning altogether.

What sort of transfer then is the Conquest Fast? It's the mightiest motor car ever occupied by man. No other vehicle is comparable to it; in adjustment, readiness, responsiveness, celerity; *cost* and *danger.* A go-cart is not conspicuously speedy, but it is reassuringly safe. The automobile record has been lowered to something less than forty seconds—but *a forty-second record means a forty-second risk.* You must be your own chauffeur. And the best in the business at that. You must know just where you're going, what road to follow, when you're likely to arrive—

and how to turn out for passers-by. You must know both the powers and limitations of your human machine. You must feel conscious control over it, measureless superiority to it. You must keep your hand on the lever, your eye on the road, and your heart on the journey's end. If you're able for it, variously able, then by all means choose this auto-motor carriage, the Conquest Fast. But—count the cost first. And don't say I promised you anything for less than the price. No one knows the price of Truth better than I; no one has paid such a price; no one would be less willing to urge the purchase on a single human soul.

RULE 2—*Analyze beforehand the errors of Popular Fasters.*

This is assuming you dare blithesomely disregard Rule One. The which I devoutly hope.

The persistent cloud on the horizon of Truth is the confusion of principle with personality. Somebody of the name of Dewey, or Macfadden, or Just, or Eddy, or Purinton, propounds a beautiful theory concerning life that may or may not be practicable. Instead of studying the *theory for ourselves,* we study the *application of the theorizer.* Which of course never fits our case. That's where all the bewilderment comes in—bewilderment dietetic, gymnastic, philosophic, therapeutic, and religious. What helps me may help you—but not in the same way it helped me. And the thing for you to do is take the truth of my principle, apart from the inevitable error of my personality. Because the automobile is a splendid vehicle is no reason for entrusting it to a raw chauffeur.

To cite details.

Not, understand, in any belittling spirit, but generously as we can. To discriminate yet not incriminate is a test for both Love and Wisdom. If sobeit possible, let us be both loving and wise. If not—let us be only loving. Rather exalt Truth because we love it than disparage error because we fear it. Not blame for others—only balance for ourselves; this should be the aim of our analysis.

The first error of the Fasting Specialist is in assuming his remedy a panacea of universal proportions. Let me say right here that the only panacea for human ills is *Understanding;* and the few rare souls that can administer this do not call themselves physicians or appraise their service in terms of money-reward. In any rational diagnosis, *temperament* is the clearest indication of both cause and cure. *Phrenology* should precede, if not supersede *Pharmacy.* I would never advise an extreme *mental* temperament to take the Conquest Fast—there must be enough of the *vital* to store energy, with enough of the *motive* to spend it. Balance is indispensable, equilibrium must be maintained. Hall Caine, for instance, would probably lose by the prolonged Fast; Alfred Henry Lewis, on the other hand, would probably gain. John D. Rockefeller is not adapted for it—he's too pious to be either vital or spiritual. Theodore Roosevelt should be a splendid subject— it would take an enforced recess to make his strenuosity subside to a comforting state of calm.

Lack of faith precludes or postpones the Conquest Fast; lack of flesh, if very pronounced; lack of vitality, in case the individual recovers it with difficulty; lack of the proper inner preparations or outer conditions; all deficiency, in short, must be considered *before* the Conquest Fast is begun. *After,* let limitations be forgot, in the larger light of dawning possibilities.

Another common error; and this is wholly physiological. Fasting is at best but a weakly negative process of cure. Its complement is *Elimination.* The waste channels of the body— bowels, kidneys, lungs and pores, should be kept peculiarly active till the latent impurities released through the Fast are brought to the surface and swept away. The mere stopping of the mechanism of digestion causes stagnation along the entire tract. So that extra precaution is required to offset this inertia. Here's a case in point. A certain hygienic healer of national reputation advised a patient to try a two-weeks' Fast. The patient acquiesced, and forthwith stopped eating. That's all—just stopped eating. Then for *nine days* the bowels failed to move. Meanwhile the man was in agony, the effect of the Fast was mostly lost, and the rightness or wrongness of the remedy could not be established in the minds of those who witnessed the perverted application. Simply because the aforesaid healer forbade all artificial stimulus to elimination—he didn't believe in massage, he thought enemas were weakening, and he deemed cathartics the Devil's ammunition. The folly of his course *seemed* to prove the folly of his theory. And so people judged.

A third common error is the failure to refer *crises* to individual *instinct*. When the time comes for decision, when the need arises for action, then must your own soul direct you—no voice from without is competent to do more than interfere. My experience cannot be yours, yours cannot be mine. The Conquest Fast always awakens a host of dormant instincts and repressed desires. Just how, no mortal can foretell. And it will be literally dangerous for you to pattern your Fast after the record of mine. Previous facts won't suffice, authentic data may not tally, reasonable expectations are likely to speed way with the wind. You are now in the hands of Nature, with your vision turned toward God. Trust both—no matter what scientific absurdities men have hitherto alleged. What cares the sun whether astronomers be peering through the peep-holes of their spy-glass? It still shines. What cares your soul whether scientists measure it or measure it not? It is still your soul. Does it not dominate forever the crude computations of these human infants not yet instructed in the multiplication-tables of divine dynamics?

A fourth common error lies in neglecting to provide against the *strain on the soul*. It is no light thing to controvert in the space of a few weeks all the habits of a lifetime and the thought-heritage of a race; you may have seen newspaper reports of people "made insane through Fasting"—through *faulty* Fasting. There must be first an *inner incentive*, second an *outer wisdom*. Forced starving is more fatal than forced stuffing—since both soul and body protest. Fasting is never to be advised as a penance—not even as a prescription. You must *want to fast more than you want to eat*, before you *can* fast with absolute safety.

Would you put out to sea in the bark canoe of a man that had never sailed before? Ere you leave the land, you must know the

Deep. And until you exert conscious guidance of your own soul, do not expect the Infinite Spirit to buoy you. It may bury you instead—the Sea does both. The psychic surge does both; witness the unsaneness of Spiritist mediums and hypnotic subjects. Not the fault of the Sea—only the deficiency of the sailor or the defect of the vessel.

RULE 3—*Get all available facts as a foundation; then forget them.*

That's all a fact is ever good for—to serve as a stone in the wall of your sub-cellar. Plant it firmly—then remember the climate is pleasanter upstairs. You should *know* all that man has discovered or proved anent Fasting—provided you don't *think* about it when you should be in the tower, watching the sunrise. Read Doctor Dewey, read Mr. Haskell, read Mr. Macfadden, read Mr. Hanish, read Mr. Shaw, read Mr. Purinton;— then smile most benignly on them all, make a cheerful bonfire of their books, and observe complaisantly how the smoke returns to the nothingness whence it came. They really don't know anything about Fasting—they're just experimenting for their own benefit.

Let me caution you moreover as to your chronology. Don't, in the name of all that's merciful, lapse into the pages of any book on Fasting *while* you are undergoing the process. That would be too much like entertaining an invalid with a picture-book of skeletons, grave-yards and scarecrows. Indeed some people are so enamored of themselves that they have their photographs taken at the end of a Fast—to show how beautiful even their bones are. Let us pass on; children can't play in a boneyard. Yet such gruesome object-lessons are more or less salutary—if anybody looked like that and lived, there's surely hope for me. The experience of others helps us only in getting our courage to the sticking-point. They did it—we can do it. They improved—we will improve. They dared be true to their beliefs, desires and intuitions—we dare be true to ours.

RULE 4—*Specify purpose and adapt regime.*

Is your chief object *Renovation, Domination, Delectation,* or *Illumination?* Which do you most want to clarify and fortify, body, brain, sense, or soul? Your answer will determine the time, the duration, the method and conditions of your Fast. Discrimination of this kind has hitherto not been made. Naturally confusion, hesitation, mistake and disappointment ensued. For instance, suppose you wish to strengthen your will-power and establish your courage beyond assault. Then decide on a certain duration—ten, twenty, or thirty days, and keep to it if the heavens fall. Suppose however you seek inspiration primarily. Then fast a day at a time; you cannot set periods and seasons for the Almighty. If your object be merely therapeutic, then a series of short Fasts will usually bring better results than a single long one. Often the adoption of a specific diet will avail more to cure disease than any Fast at all. Especially as few people are free to leave their home or their business for any length of time. If you work you must eat—and some of us feel rather obliged to work—in order that we may eat! Such an endless chain of folly.

I have been asked this question:

"How can the average wife and mother manage a Conquest Fast, with her husband, her children, her household and her social duties to consider?"

My answer is prompt and concise—"She can't."

She'll be doing well if she gets her husband educated up to the Two-Meal Plan, with no company for dinner. In the matter of eating, there is only one creature on earth more absurd than the society woman. That creature is the business man. He doesn't know it—he doesn't know much of anything really worth knowing. And if you told him, he would proceed to disprove it with a new lot of glib fallacies fresh-fashioned for the occasion. I hope some day to write a book on "Man Irrational." He's unquestionably the queerest animal extant—as a species and as a sex. Certainly no ornithologist has yet done him justice.

But in the home where Love rules—and there is no home elsewhere—every member of the family may do as that member pleases. Comings and goings are unrestricted, thoughts and acts pass unchallenged. Moreover, when one is quite ready in one's own soul for the Conquest Fast, the way will always open. It is our fear that limits us—not our faith. Faith leads us on and out and up, so far and so fast as we dare follow.

A good deal depends on the character of our work, whether at home or in the office. If it be very exacting for brain or body, we had best omit, or postpone, or modify the extreme Fast. Though I have known active business men to labor incessantly through twenty, thirty, even forty days' abstention from food. Here again the temperament and attitude of mind must direct.

In a word; read these Rules in the light of your own desire. Apply them so far as you deem them sane and opportune;—break them, refute them, transcend them in whatever respect Love and Truth sanction.

RULE 5—*Choose Summer or Spring for the Conquest Fast.*
There are at least four reasons.

First: fresh fruits and vegetables may be had before and after the Fast. Nothing takes the place of the salts and juices obtained fresh in our garden products; both in preparing the body for active elimination and in helping it recover tone. Either canning or drying vitiates the nourishing elements. So the season when green things grow is by far the best for any change in dietetic regime.

Second: the temperature and atmospheric conditions favor purification. You can perspire freely without special effort—a vital point in the physiology of Fasting. In cool weather recourse must be had to Turkish, vapor or hot-air baths; measures more or less unnatural and unquestionably enervating. Sun-baths, moreover, are as indispensable to restore vitality as to quicken elimination; sun-baths in winter being almost nil.

Third: the accustomed inertia of the season makes idling easier. Spring fever is so much the fashion, summer ennui so altogether proper, that the Fast won't violate our conventional code of morals and manners in the effect it produces on our activities. Not an ounce of energy should be dissipated during the extreme Fast. It is enough to burn out the waste; whatever is good flesh and blood must be conserved to produce more. This means loafing, resting, lazing along and not caring. Evidently a summer programme.

Fourth: the gala garb of Nature attracts us to the open. You can't take a Conquest Fast in the house—would you try to swim in a barrel? Expanse is the first possession required by the soul in the process of freeing itself. Out and away from the mortal, on and up into the consciousness of the Eternal; thus shall the soul advance. Even through the heat of summer you will find the clouds quite cold enough—no need to add the bareness of the earth and the bleakness of the sky in winter. At best the Conquest Fast is a crucial ordeal; let us make the conditions as comfortable as we can without compromise.

RULE 6—*Prepare for the long Fast by the experience of a few short ones.*

Otherwise you might think you were going to die the second day. Not a pleasing prospect—with twenty or thirty more to-morrows like it coming in a string. Fasts of from one to three days or longer concluded safely may embolden those who haven't the nerve for a month-stretch at first. Say live a week without food, in April or May, if you plan a month's Fast for July or August. This precaution is mostly for timid souls—brave ones will scorn it. I never fasted a day voluntarily until I quit food for a month—couldn't brook any props or palliatives, wanted the very hardest feat in spiritual gymnastics that any soul ever attempted. But the sinews of my soul were strong. I could face hazard with a smile. I had wrested victory from defeat. I knew my powers, I recognized my limitations. So that what would be ominous and perilous for most mortals had become simple and natural for me. The harder the struggle, the greater the triumph. Judge for yourself how strong you are.

RULE 7—*Plan work congenial but not compulsory.*

This on the supposition that you cannot afford to be wholly idle, or that you have not learned to relax utterly. During the Fast, nothing should drive you save the impulse of your own soul, nothing direct you save the Voice of the Infinite. Work as you want to, play as you want to, read as you want to, rest as you want to, dream as you want to. At the start you are likely to have severe headaches; off and on you may be subject to attacks of weakness or faintness; nothing serious, still inconvenient. You may find it harder to sleep through the night, but easier to nap by day. Then there is the pestilence of personality to be considered. Living as common humans do, you may have escaped—on the homeopathic principle of "Like cure like." But when you have clarified your immortal Self from your earthy tendencies, you notice all at once how insufferably gross the people around you are become. And if your work compels you to mingle with them, you can't fast long without suffocating. Keep occupied if you will—but let it be happily so. Under no circumstances attempt a Conquest Fast while subject to the rules, orders and suspicions of the average employer. You will lose more than you gain.

RULE 8—*Be alone, or among strangers.*

The surest way to make a man your enemy is to give him plenty of "friendly advice." On this assumption, every friend of the man on a Fast becomes his direst foe. If they don't worry themselves into hysterics for fear you'll starve to death, they will at least comment on your looks, diagnose your symptoms, ask you to describe your feelings, in short plague clean out of you the very life they are so solicitous to preserve. No optician ever found spectacles to relieve the short-sightedness of Solicitude; it's congenital and can't be cured.

Don't even tell your friends and relatives you expect to fast. Unless perchance you be blessed with that rare gift of the gods— a comrade or a sweetheart who understands. The comfort to be had from the counsel and sympathy of this One would be quite legitimate and unspeakably reassuring. Go out camping; hire a house-boat; get lodgings at some distant farmer's, coming in only at night; best of all, roll up a few accessories in a staunch sleeping-bag and hie you to some solitary spot amid the mountains or by the sea-shore.

Another reason besides the interference of friends. If you are daily associating with people addicted to the three-meal monotony, you can't help seeing, smelling, and remembering food. Not a salutary situation for one trying so desperately to forget food. Keep away from the table, the cupboard, the cook-book and the dinner-bell. Not because you might be "tempted to eat" —in that case, stick right there till you've conquered the errant tendency. But because you are living on a higher plane and must not be irritated by such coarse vibrations as eating sets in motion.

Still a third consideration. Complete change of scene is essention to the vantage of a new perspective. No trace of old relationships, no iteration of memory's bidding, no diverting influence should be suffered to interpose between you and the horizon. Any psychometrist will tell you how completely inanimate objects are invested with the aura of their owners or users. Books, pictures, furniture, what not—all bear a message of good or ill that we must receive whether we will or not. The very air of a leprous house is a curse, the very atmosphere of a place of worship is a benediction. All of which serves to emphasize the necessity for being alone while achieving the Fast.

Rule 9—*Keep near Nature.*

A smile and a pair of sandals is quite sufficient clothing— you don't really need the sandals. Take all the sun-baths consistent with comfort, and an occasional clay compress (for directions, see Adolph Just's "Return to Nature"). Lie flat on the earth as much as you can. Dabble in the brook, or play in the waves of the sea. Get used to sleeping on the grass; indeed some folks are such strenuous Naturists they dig up the sod and bury themselves over night in the bare soil. Sounds kind of clammy, doesn't it? 'Tisn't necessary—except to try. Find how much nourishment Nature provides that isn't called food. The fragrance of the forest and aroma of the wild is sustaining; the breath of the breeze exhilarates; the thrill of the earth-contact vivifies; the glance of the sun both soothes and empowers. Provender for the stomach takes a minor place in the economy of human life, when once provision for the soul has been made independently.

RULE 10—*Avoid combinations with other systems of Naturopathy.*

The Conquest Fast doesn't harmonize with the Kneipp Water Cure, or the Macfadden School of Physical Culture, or any other regime that demands large expenditure of energy and vitality. These methods may be ever so good—they are not timely.

I knew of a man that had chronic rheumatism. He consulted a Fasting-specialist;—and stopped eating. Began to feel better, wondered if he couldn't be improving faster. Consulted a Turkish Bath-specialist;—and began bathing. Presently he died. Then each specialist declared the other killed the patient. They were both doctors, too, with a national reputation and a big sanitarium to back it. Fasting *alone* might have healed the sufferer— *or* Baths alone. Together they took out more vitality than virus, leaving him clean no doubt—a clean corpse. Doubtless a Theosophist would gain some consolation from the thought of how pure his body was when he left it. But to those of us not of the elect it looks like a plain case of malpractice.

Don't turn your ambition toward any "stunts" of physical prowess, after the first week of a long Fast. It's the time to store energy—not to spend it. If you never learned how to let things slide, this is your opportunity supreme. Both materially and spiritually, repose must be reckoned a chief component in the Conquest Fast.

RULE 11—*The week preceding the Fast, let your diet be wholly laxative.*

This to correct the invariable tendency to stoppage noticed the first few days of a Fast. Not only should there be no residue of waste matter to be eliminated when the mechanism of digestion has ceased; but the excretory functions should be specially active for the arousing and expelling of the latent impurities dragged from their hiding by the Fast. Fresh fruits and vegetables, with a few nuts and crisp cereals; let these form the mainstay for the week preceding. Care also is advisable in the matter of mastication—see the books by Horace Fletcher for elaboration of this subject. Since intestinal stagnation is due mostly to unchewed and therefore undigested particles of food on which the bowel juices cannot act. Lessening the variety at each meal may be advantageous—he who eats too fast and he who eats too much being one and the same person.

RULE 12—*Think of something besides Fasting.*

That is, if you have to think at all. It's better to stop thinking altogether. Dream instead. If you can't dream, at least you can doze. Anything to make that obstreporous brain of yours be still, until your soul has spoken. Now, if ever, may you vault the earthly limitations of the human mind, to roam where you will through the sunlit chambers of the Limitless. Indeed to think of eating is to invite nausea. Since the very concept of food is distasteful so long as an atom of impurity remains in the body. We are usually so bound in the thrall of habit-hunger as not to notice whether we enjoy the meal. Once stop all this, and forthwith the unassimilated particles from years of rash eating are transformed into gas or liquid, to cloud the brain, coat the tongue, clog the blood and chafe the palate. We won't be hungry till the situation clears. And we haven't any business to think about food except when we are hungry.

Let me commend first and foremost the ministry of Music. Nothing takes us so quickly out of our earth-environment, nothing puts us so fully en rapport with the rhapsodies of angels. Sing as you never sang before. Play whatever instrument comes easiest and expresses most. Listen outside the church door for the Organ Voluntary (I don't prescribe the Anthem or the Hymns). If there be melody in a baby's prattle, or harmony in a woman's murmur—let this move you. Above all, may your senses be attuned to the celestial symphony of sea and hills, sun and stars, all resonant with the choral chime of Nature's host.

Then there are books of special import. Works of Poetry, Invention, Discovery, and Philosophy head the list. Emerson, Whitman, Browning, Thoreau, Goethe, Wordsworth; take some of these with you into retirement. Elbert Hubbard's "Little Journeys" would be not inopportune; perhaps also literature of direct tonic value might appeal; say Thomson J. Hudson's "Law of Mental Medicine," or Herbert A. Parkyn's "Auto-Suggestion," or Annie Payson Call's "Power through Repose," or Ralph Waldo Trine's "In Tune with the Infinite." Whatever book can enlarge your horizon, refine your sympathies, strengthen your faith and inspire your soul—this is the book to read while you fast.

RULE 13—*Devote the first three days to special elimination.*

That is, stimulate bowels, kidneys, lungs and pores to do double service. Fully half the benefit of the extreme Fast is lost if impurities be allowed to remain in the body in excess of the body's capacity to expel them. Vapor-baths are therefore in order (you can buy a good cabinet for $5); enemas; deep breathing exercises; abdominal massage; copious water drinking—hot unsweetened lemonade is most efficacious; friction baths; perhaps a single stomach lavage; even a dose of liver pills in case the colon flushing falls short of the stoppage.

I should say in general a vapor-bath would be advisable the first and third day; an enema daily for a week; a thorough friction bath every morning; an abdominal or general massage each afternoon; a long walk in the evening with all the exhilaration you can get out of deep, slow, rhythmic, peaceful breathing. Drink at least two quarts of water during the day, preferably a half-glass at a time. Acid fruit-juice cannot be surpassed as an aid to elimination—about a half a glass for the twenty-four hours, well diluted with perhaps three times its bulk of water. Orange-juice is best, with lemon-juice and grape-juice close seconds. Nor is pineapple, cherry, or lime forbidden. If you are fasting principally for *Illumination*, you can't be haunted with the memory

or irritated by the taste of even fruit-juice. But for clarifying
of brain and body, a little of this may be taken through most of
the Fast—one kind only, in order not to indulge the palate. There
is a trifle nourishment in grape-juice, hence the orange seems better suited to the needs of the Faster. Lemon is too stringent for
steady use.

After I had received the vision I sought through the Fast,
I began taking fruit-juice in small quantities. It quieted the
stomach, soothed the nerves, cleared the tongue and the brain,
especially acted as a laxative. For with me a most unusual experience ensued—the bowels moved freely, once during the third
week of the Fast, once during the fourth. Due unquestionably to
the influence of the fruit-juice.

Indeed for a short Fast, any under ten days, I would suggest the moderate use of the orange, lemon or grape—carefully re-
jecting all the pulp. Such recourse allays fermentation, dispels
noxious gases, assists elimination, hastens purification, and lessens
the mental strain of rupturing suddenly the eating-habit fastened
on the race. The juice of three oranges a day should be sufficient.

RULE 14—*Use water plentifully but gently.*

You may walk in the dew with Father Kneipp—you may not
follow him to the extremes of the "Blitzguss." A Priessnitz
Compress daily, a Just or Kuhne Bath, a tepid shower—some
such measure as this, in preference to the cold plunge or douche.
No shock should be permitted, no vitality wasted.

As to the amount of water taken internally, opinions differ.
Instinct, here as always, may be assumed the only safe guide. In
general we may say however, that the one occasion when instinct
might be forced is in the matter of water-drinking during a Fast.
Cultivate a desire for it. Drink not less than a glass an hour
on the average, unless you feel discomfort or repulsion therefrom. Of course if you have suffered from dilated stomach or
impaired kidneys, the amount may well be lessened. Mountain
spring-water is the best. But it must be pure and it must be soft.

Otherwise let the variety be distilled and aerated. Bottled spring-water may be substituted if you are sure of its analysis.

RULE 15—*Let treatment be passive rather than active.*
This on the assumption that you're still in the "treatment" stage, or that the therapeutic purpose is uppermost. During the extreme Fast is the only time I would suggest any such dependence on people or things outside oneself. But then it is entirely to be commended. If you know a good mental or magnetic healer, let him exercise his gifts without let or hindrance—even though he employ such crude measures as passes, manipulations, suggestions, vibrations, or "affirmations." Massage is clearly indicated, especially spinal and abdominal. Get all the sleep you can, by night and day both. A specialist in health-hypnotics or post-hypnotic suggestion might be employed to advantage, in assuring slumber and also quietude for the waking hours. Even so unscientific a practitioner as a Christian Science devotee could be called in to help establish faith and prepare the way for soul certitude. But don't tell the Christian Science sister you're fasting—she doesn't believe in that. Jesus fasted, Jesus used hydrotherapy, psychology, "malicious animal magnetism," and other natural influences in his marvels of healing. Jesus was a Naturist no less than a mystic. Yet the vital side of the Nazarene has been repudiated by the Christian Scientists; that's why they call themselves "Christian"—they want to be but can't.

Vigorous action required by games, gymnastics and the like should be limited to the first few days of the Conquest Fast. After that, leisurely walking is in order, together with gentle *stretching* movements and *breathing* exercises. A Fast of only a week or so would not be sufficiently devitalizing to preclude muscular effort throughout. In general, nothing that takes initiative, whether of body, brain or soul, should be planned for the period of the Fast. Omnipotence is working—let the mortal retire.

RULE 16—*Focus on local troubles.*
We call them "troubles"—until we make them triumphs.

Any disorder, physical or mental, may be reached with thrice the despatch and efficacy during an extreme Fast. The system has been cleared of both irritating impurities and conflicting vibrations, all the vital forces are ready to respond to a given appeal at a given point, Nature's inherent tendency toward recuperation exhibits a peculiar urgency and a gratifying swiftness.

If, for instance, the liver seems torpid constitutionally, now is the time to wake it up. With hot fomentations, cold douches and compresses, earth-packs, strong massage, deep breathing together with bending and twisting movements, mental treatments, and whatever else may serve a similar purpose.

Nervous dyspepsia, heart disease, bronchial ailments, mental derangements, and various other inharmonies seem specially to respond to the right healing influences exerted during a Fast. Nature unaided will cure everything in time, if we only give her a chance. But it sort of assures us to think we're helping along, besides relieving the unusual strain of mental vacuity. No— brains aren't too empty as it is! They're stuffed, hopelessly stuffed with facts they can't digest, assimilate and work over into life. If brains were oftener vacant, minds would be sooner filled.

Rule 17—*Learn to laugh at symptoms.*

Also at the silly folk who note symptoms. While we're speaking of people, let me call your attention to the absurd appearance of them that have to eat. Feeding one's face is a grotesque operation at best. But when humans actually make it the basis for all sociability, hospitality, fellowship and good cheer—the performance is so ridiculous as to be pathetic. Poke barrels of fun at the family while they bow their knee to the cook. Observe how closely their gastronomic gyration resembles the munching of their simian brethren. Over the meal's digestibility assume an air of dubiety and a prophecy of colic that'll make them wish stomachs were never invented. Let them see you're It—while they? They are a sort of raw hash, half-remnant, half-rudiment. Remnant of what a good animal might have been, rudiment of what a passable man may become in time. It's so common, so vulgar, so insufferably plebeian to have to eat; you belong to a superior race of beings that eat only when they choose to. Just now you don't choose—and it's such fun to lord it over the minion Knights of the Knife-and-fork.

But we started to say something about symptoms. That reminds us of doctors—dim pallid memory. A doctor thinks it his duty to give so many drugs because he takes so many symptoms —on the principle, I suppose, that fair exchange of foul deeds is no robbery. A doctor's absurdity is equalled only by his solemnity—and his whiskers, these being the limit of both. There is nothing in the long catalogue of drug-school fallacies so unscientific as an isolated symptom. It tells nothing and foretells less. It's the single flicker of a moving-picture machine that started a generation back and must run till a generation hence. If you want Truth, don't bother with symptoms. Watch principles and examine causes—actions and results can look out for themselves.

Here's a case in point. Lots of people say that fresh fruit "disagrees" with them. It doesn't. It can't. They "disagree" with themselves. Their stomachs are so full of undigested food that the acid of the fruit stirs up a ferment from the midst of the decay. The morbid matter must be got out somehow—the fruit says anyhow. But the stupid eater answers "No, let the stuff stay so long as I don't know it's there." Then the doctor takes his hush-money to keep the ferment silenced—and it's "cut out fruit." Dope the symptom to cure the disease; that's the highly rational theory of the highly scientific drug-dispenser.

Now during the long Fast you'll lose a lot of weight—probably an average of a pound a day. Never mind—it's a good riddance of bad rubbish. You'll get it all back at the close of the Fast, with an increase of perhaps a pound and a half a day; and this time it will be pure blood, firm flesh, sound sinew. You may feel unaccountably weak, strangely insecure. No need to worry—it's mostly imagination. Physiologically there should be no real loss of strength till *brain, nerve and muscle* actually waste away; which never occurs while an ounce of flesh remains to be oxygenized. Often a sensation akin to weakness accompanies the passage of impurities from the body—brain, blood, bowels, lungs, kidneys, pores, all are serving as special sewer-functions at the beginning of a Fast. And since the waste matter in process of decay always leaves first, the initial part of the Fast is naturally the most uncomfortable. As a matter of fact, *the worse you feel, the better you are.* Rather, the better becoming—you wouldn't *feel* bad now if you hadn't *been* bad for a long time before. This is what Naturopaths call the "crisis," the expulsion to the surface and appearance thereon of all the foulness lurking deep in the system perhaps for half a lifetime. So that the more miserable you feel, the more certain is your need for a Fast. The quickest way to make a Freethinker believe in Hell is to put him on a long Fast; he'll be there the first week. But the third or fourth week he'll arrive at Heaven—so he won't hold a grudge against you. There's no place in Heaven to hide a grudge—too much sunshine everywhere. Suggestion to theologues; the "bottomless pit" is the pit of the stomach—span that and you're saved.

Flabby and anaemic women in particular will find themselves "all gone," perhaps haunted by a choice array of fears, dreads and phantoms. Don't be alarmed—it's only the ghosts of those sickly Charlotte Russes making their departure. Maybe some Sally Lunns are buried there too. Might as well dig up the whole cemetery while you're about it—so flowers can grow there next spring. Remember all the while that the Fast is not to blame; rather the folly that preceded and necessitated the Fast. And be glad you're getting some sense at last, even if it does cost a pain or two.

Your pulse may drop twenty degrees—one I knew went from 86 to 68 in four days. Sudden attacks of dizziness, vertigo, and the like may annoy you, especially on rising quickly. Headaches of a variegated assortment may follow themselves in motley caravan. A hundred and one unsuspected conditions may develop sooner or later. Again I say—"Laugh at symptoms—pooh-pooh them out of business." You are more momentous than your feels-ifs. And so long as you know you are right—to Halifax with the bogie mob. I'd say "to Hell," but I'm very careful about offending "members of the cloth." How that describes them—tailor's dummies of Theology.

RULE 18—*Wait and trust for results.*

The finest things are always the most impalpable. A man feels pain, a child feels pleasure, but only a mother feels the ecstacy of anguish. For only a mother is attuned to both earth and heaven.

It takes eons of evolution to unfold a mother-soul. And you can't expect to feel all the glories of being after a few days or weeks of soul-stirring. *Not during the Fast* do you notice great improvement—rather when the Fast is over and forgotten. But I assure you there will ensue such a degree of rejuvenation as will atone for every moment of suffering, every particle of discomfort. Especially on the higher planes of perception.

I spent a few weeks in the country last summer, profiting by the lessons learned through Fasting. While living in the open, scarce a single direct inspiration came to me. But in the month following my return to town, I wrote a *hundred and twenty-five new poems.* Consciousness gathers somewhat as a cloud—slowly, silently, imperceptibly. But when it breaks, then the world knows you have been on the summit of aspiration, breathing in the mists.

RULE 19—*Break the Fast with a morsel and a prayer.*

The crux of a long Fast is the breaking of it. Returning to the world seems even harder than leaving it. For a week or so in transition you must be half animal with the animal's unerring instinct, half mystic with the mystic's unwavering ideal, not at all man with the man's hesitancy, temptation and defeat. You will be very empty indeed when you begin to eat again—but by that time you should have learned to enjoy being empty. The stomach won't call for a third the food the rest of you seems to demand. Because the stomach has grown weak from enforced inaction, the digestive juices have lent themselves in other directions, the entire machinery of assimilation is too quiet to disturb by any shock of sudden imposition.

A single article is enough for the first meal, two will suffice for the second, three for the third, fourth, fifth and sixth. Eat whatever you crave most, spend at least an hour in masticating, enjoying and idealizing. Then wait six hours before you taste food again. Among the best Fast-breaking selections let me offer these: *Popcorn, Toasted Triscuit, Lust's Whole Wheat Zwieback,* an *apple,* two or three dried *peaches or prunes,* a small saucer of *whole wheat* boiled and baked in its own juice, *a piece* of crusty *corn-bread,* or a cup of thick *pea soup.* Something in short that requires mastication and furnishes sufficient fibre to act on the intestinal walls. I broke my Fast on a saucer of toasted wheat. It took 700 chews to liquefy the first spoonful, and nearly 40 minutes to complete the dish. A really hungry mortal can't bolt his food—it's a physiological impossibility. And he doesn't need half so much to satisfy him, because he digests and uses all that enters the stomach. Most people's digestion is so torpid they can't get good from more than a small fraction of what they eat; hence the unbalanced aspect of their diet, in both choice and amount. This explains the dulness and depression so often felt after meals—just the protest of an overworked and enfeebled stomach calling for more than its share of blood to perform what should be a joy instead of a perfunctory duty.

You will not need or desire more than half the habitual rations consumed before the Fast—provided of course you follow instinct absolutely in the choice, amount, duration and mental attitude respecting food and meal-time. I said "with a morsel and a prayer." By that I don't mean you should "say a blessing." Rather, feel a consecration. Your horizon-view should have clarified some great purpose for your living, some beautiful ideal for your attaining. Keep this in mind while you partake of the material nourishment that enables your soul to express its message on earth. Vision a halo over every morsel. See your heart's sublimest hope realizing though the power from the food.

Eat with the joy of an animal, love with the consciousness of a god.

RULE 20—*Expect ensuing change in life.*

Even a week's Fast has opened a new perspective to the individual who took it. You observe a distinct vantage, in realms of body, mind, heart and soul. Things don't look as they used to. The real seems real where before it appeared vague. The false, the unnatural, the superfluous and the unlovely all retire into the shadow of oblivion where they belong. Henceforth you are yourself and the world is nothing. You know naught but that Truth beckons and Love empowers. You have severed the old bonds, formed before you knew yourself or dared be true. You have passed through a new birth, you are living in the Heaven of Sincerity. You may find the world does not recognize you but treats you as an alien. Old friends may desert you—new friends shall cherish you. Habits, customs, desires, ambitions, thoughts, feelings, lovings—all are subject to change under the transforming power of the Conquest Fast.

But the Eternal does not waver, nor the Infinite diminish. You can well afford to emerge from the haze of humanity, wherein men saw you dimly and grasped for you feebly;—out—on—up—into the splendor of Divinity, whence men flee your glory and leave you alone with God.

AN INDIVIDUAL EPILOGUE

As an improvement over a "Personal Prologue."

The Prologue was a recital of symptoms, of surroundings, of limitations and deficiencies, of imperfections and unattained longings.

The Epilogue is an assertion of Self.

It took what wasn't I some twenty-two years to get through with the Prologue. It has taken Me five years to arrive at so much of the Epilogue as is here recorded. I haven't got very far yet en route for Truth. But you may observe the difference in speed when a personality follows the crowd and when an individual starts forth for itself.

Personality is the envy of small souls—and the bane of great ones.

Individuality is the terror of small souls—and the glory of great ones.

I have called the Epilogue "A Declaration of Faith."

NOT a "Confession." I do not apologize for my belief. I exult in it. And I yearn over any soul that has not one of equal proportions.

It is fitting that Faith should supply the last word. Because in the end of all things, matter melts to mystery; Science halts dumb in the presence of Religion; Logic steps aside to make way for Love; Mind turns back to its earth-environ, and only Spirit soars on untrammeled to explore and accredit the unlogical, undemonstrable, undebatable certitudes of the Almighty.

A DECLARATION OF FAITH

I believe.

I believe in believing.

I believe that, next to loving, believing is wisest and most Godlike.

I believe that the good of believing lies in the believing—not in the belief.

I believe that your belief is none of my business.

I believe that the belief of to-day may be unbelievable to-morrow, and needn't feel ashamed either.

I believe that depth of belief without breadth is more desirable than breadth without depth.

I believe that the absolute belief of the child may and should accompany the absolute knowledge of the man.

I believe that Faith and Fact are not foes but friends—when each recognizes and respects the province of the other.

I believe, however, that a blind belief is better than no belief.

I believe that so long as a man's belief satisfies him, it is an unkindness to shake it, whether by reform, pessimism, or proselytism.

I believe that the only way to justify a belief is to keep silent concerning it; and the only way to prove it is to live it.

I believe that belief in Self is the highest form of belief—and the rarest.

———

I believe in myself.

I believe in you.

I believe in everybody and everything.

I believe in the undiminishable purity, sweetness, and strength of the human soul.

I believe in the Fatherhood, Motherhood, and Babyhood of God.

I believe in the gentleness of Justice and the far-sightedness of Fate.

I believe in an all-pervasive Omniscience-Omnipotence, competent to deify any soul that trusts It.

I believe in the wisdom that masters the intricacies of occult science—and the greater wisdom that forgets them.

I believe in miracles that cease to be miracles when one knows the Law.

I believe in the Bible—as the repository of the most and the best beliefs.

I believe in Jesus as his own divine savior—and in Me as mine.

I believe in the unchurched and unconfined Christ resident potential in every incarnate soul.

I believe in the religion of kindness, thoughtfulness, courage, cheerfulness, and brotherly love.

I believe in the charity never called by that name.

I believe in the dignity of labor, the joy of work, the sweetness of rest, and the satisfaction of symmetry.

I believe in the sacredness of the human body; and I shudder at the blasphemy of such as would hide it, bind it, abuse it, misrepresent it, or call it impure.

I believe in the majesty, beauty, divinity, and ecstacy of Sex.

I believe in a man's motherhood and a woman's brotherhood.

I believe in the home where Love is—and no other.

I believe in the divorce where Love is not—and no other.

I believe in the avowed sinner more than in the avowed saint.

I believe in the penalty that none save Nature inflicts.

I believe in suffering as a refining process; and in the exquisite anguish of soul-travail.

I believe in the immortality of my soul; therefore it matters not whether my name become immortal.

I believe in both the dreams of the idealist and the deeds of the materialist; impression heavenward with expression earthward.

I believe in the hope that every man has for himself; my hope being world-wide and eternity-long.

I believe in a Consciousness that transcends the mortal; emerging from the mists of time, place, person and circumstance, till it melts clear and pure into the effulgence of the Most High.

I believe that the world needs me.

I believe that the world will reward me richly—when I deserve recompense.

I believe that my poverty is nobody's fault but my own; therefore am I not a Socialist.

I believe that my neighbor treats me as I treat him—or a little better; so I hold no grudge against anybody.

I believe that my expression of belief helps me most; I am not concerned if nobody listens.

I believe that the only way I can be faithful to you is to be faithful to myself.

I believe that my only duty is to know and follow my desire.

I believe that the Infinite is none too large for me to aspire to.

I believe that countless eons have heaped themselves that I may lord them all; and I do.

I believe that reform is as unwise as it is unavailing.

I believe that polemics are futile if not fatal.

I believe that criticism is a confession of impotence; since the critic is never the creator.

I believe that codes of conduct are for cowards only.

I believe that law-breakers are nearer right than law-makers.

I believe that the crimes against criminals are the cruelest of all.

I believe that the only sin is shutting one's eyes to the light in one's own soul.

I believe that consistency is either lethargy or hypocrisy.

I believe that Instinct is infallible—so far as not yet paralyzed by civilization.

I believe that every man is part animal and part angel; if he be a man, he is neither ashamed of the one nor afraid of the other.

I believe that life is more valuable than learning; and the day-laborer a truer counsellor than the college professor.

I believe that there is no arrogance so haughty and so cruel as the pride of mentality.

I believe that in general the more one knows the more one misunderstands.

I believe that Truth is indivisible and illimitable, being neither scientific, religious, philosophical, commercial or sentimental.

I believe that Science and Religion were born sisters, but that Superstition has parted them for the time being.

I believe that in scientific parenthood lies the salvation of the race; but Science must not dictate to Love.

I believe that Humanity is constantly improving; perhaps in a million ages it may be presentable.

I believe that the only devil is the dread of our weaker mortality; and the only hell that sense of suffocation attending an earth-aura.

I believe that Heaven is here and now in the hearts of the heavenly-minded; but that greater splendors transcending human imagination await us on the other side.

I believe that Death is an angel of light, ushering the soul into a brighter palace of Possibility; and if our vision were fine enough, we could always catch a glimpse of glory as the portal swings open.

I believe that the Millennium comes to each soul individually, marking the close of this earth-school of experience and the Commencement Day in a larger sphere.

I believe that these beliefs and whatever truer may ensue will forever pale into nothingness beside the one thing

I KNOW—

That Love Alone Suffices.

APPENDIX

(Of Interest to those who Believe more or less in the Book)

IF YOU STILL EAT

—why not make the operation as pleasant and safe as possible?

Most hygienic eating is **harmless** enough—if only it were **painless!**

Nothing can be better than it tastes—whether it's food, medicine, reform, ethics, law, or theology. And if you don't like a thing it can't be good for you. This isn't saying you will like all at once whatever is best for you—people's likes and dislikes usually have to be straightened out before they can tell just what they do want.

Naturopaths don't believe in peptonized sawdust—except for chickens. Nor in predigested near-food—except for babes in their first or second childhood. Nutriment that is natural is **both wholesome and palatable**—and you don't often find it.

Do you enjoy a Good Dinner? Or are you considering a Long Fast? Then in either case you need to know about the Naturopathic Health Store, 124 East 59th Street, City of New York. The best foods to introduce the Fast as well as to break it are there waiting for you. And the man in charge can tell you more about Natural Diet in ten minutes than you could learn from books in a month.

Here are some of the specialties you'll discover at this Store: Whole Wheat Bread, Crackers and Zwieback (fresh, sweet and crispy); Nut Butter (suits some folks better than dairy butter, costs less and keeps forever); Kneipp Malt Coffee (known the world over as the only **real** equivalent of ordinary coffee with the caffein in); Plasmon, Tropon, Strengthening Soup and other invalids' foods; Imported German Chocolates, Beverages and various products you have to taste to appreciate; **Honest** Cereals, both the newest and best; Special Combinations of Nuts with Fruits that many people say they can't do without; and lots more good things for the sick and well, young and old, good, bad and indifferent.

If you live nearby, or ever pass through the city, why not try a Naturopathic Dinner at the Naturopathic Health Home? Same address as Store—upstairs. You'll get a new idea of hygienic eating, one not presented elsewhere in this country.

Vegetarian, Raw Food and Naturopathic Cook Books on sale at the Store. Save money, time, drudgery, temper and doctors' bills.

Somewhere in *The Philosophy of Fasting* the best garb is declared to be "a smile and a pair of sandals." Both to be had at the Naturopathic Store—sell the sandals and give away the smile. Be sure you get the smile anyway.

Everything else kept that helps toward natural healing and living. Bath Cabinets and Appliances; Linen-Mesh Porous Underwear; Imported Soaps that both cleanse, soothe and heal; Kneipp Herbal Remedies and Preparations; Physical Culture Supplies, Exercisers and Equipment; Books, Charts and Pamphlets on Hydrotherapy, Massage,

Rational Diet, Gymnastics, Strength and Beauty Culture, Deep Breathing, New Thought, Mental Science, Suggestion, Will Power and Soul Unfoldment.

This is news—not advertising.

So prices aren't given.

But lists and catalogues would be forthcoming if you asked for them. Might enclose a stamp or two by way of courtesy. Mark your letter "Personal to Mr. Lust" and get a reply direct to all your questions—if you have any.

N.B.—Don't take the Health problem too seriously. Children who work over their "sums" when it is time to go out and play may expect to have a headache. If that's you—why take a recess. Laugh and forget—you'll see clearer when you come back to your study of Life.

THINKING ISN'T ALWAYS FATAL

—though you might infer so from the trend of certain passages in this Book.

A little boy has to cut himself before he learns how to whittle; but he isn't likely to inflict serious damage if you keep him well supplied with pine sticks to hack at. The human brain is like a sharp jack-knife in the hands of a rash child—it's sure to cut him before he discovers what it's for. The best you can do is to ask him please make you a cane, or a flower-trellis, or a willow whistle—and so keep the youngster from amputating his own fingers by way of enjoying himself.

We can't think too much—we can feel too little; we can't philosophize too much—we can love too little; we can't learn too much—we can live too little. To live as fast as we learn—this is the criterion for the value of our learning. Success is but knowing and doing some one thing better than anybody else knows it or does it.

And so Naturopathy says "Read little—practise much." We do not advise the perusal of many books on Health, Saneness and Happiness. Rather the mastery of a few. Indeed the entire theory and practice of "Return to Nature" is presented quite adequately in three works—those of Bilz, Kneipp and Just. Thousands of sufferers from all sorts of chronic disease have been healed permanently by each of these systems. So that a word of description seems not out of place.

1. "The Natural Method of Healing" by F. E. Bilz, the famous physician of Dresden, Germany, is the most comprehensive work ever published in any language on a similar subject. Gives results of many years' experience in a successful sanitarium, enabling anybody to heal himself at home by the same methods. Explains and exemplifies Sun, Light, Air and Diet Cure, Gymnastics and Physical Culture, Hydrotherapy in all its branches, Massage, Magnetic Healing, Manipulations, Lung Culture, Care of the Sick, Special and Exclusive Information for Nurses, Doctors and Naturopaths—a complete compendium, in short, of the entire Naturopathic School of Practice. 2,600 pages, 700 pages, 30 colored charts and plates. A million copies already sold in Europe—where whole families use it as a Handbook of Health. Diseases and Cures indexed alphabetically, described accurately and proven authen-

tic by actual cases—hundreds of them. This is the **one book indispensable** to every human interested in his own health, its recovery or preservation.

2. **"The Water-Cure,"** by Sebastian Kneipp, tells just how the author cured the ailments of himself and then thousands more by the simple use of Water and a few Herbs. Kneipp was perhaps the most renowned Natural Healer that ever lived—certainly he treated the most patients and cured the worst cases. As many as 2,000 persons at one time have been under his instructions and ministrations. This book gives the story of his life and success. For simple treatment and quick results in all forms of chronic disease, the Water-Cure stands unrivalled. And Kneipp is the world's recognized authority on the subject.

3. **"Return to Nature,"** by Adolf Just, has already been referred to in various sections of this Book. The works of Bilz and Kneipp deal directly with the **practice of Natural Healing**—that of Just treats more of the **principles of Natural Living.** How to become perfect animals —that is his theme. And yet he so links body with soul as to make his belief in poetry, idealism, and heart-sympathy seem the natural complement of his Nut and Fruit Diet, Air Baths, and Earth Applications. Just has the typical American temperament—nervous, intense, with the mental and digestive tendency to disease so prevalent in our cities. So the record of his personal triumph over so-called "incurable" afflictions should and does interest Twentieth Century Americans especially. This book gives the clearest **insight into the reason and rationale** of Naturism of any yet issued.

Don't think too long about whether you want these treatises or not—just sit down now and write for circulars, for explicit information and convincing proofs. Address Naturopathic Publishing Company, 124 East 59th Street, New York City, and say where you saw the announcement.

"Everything in Nature Cure and Advanced Thought"—that describes the scope of this concern. So you needn't be bashful about asking questions or saying you want things—it's Naturopathy's business to meet you more than half-way. Would come all the way, only the exercise will do you good.

P.S.—If you aren't too tired thinking, there's a magazine called "Naturopath" that some people consider worth reading last month, this month and next. Mr. Lust edits it, Mr. Purinton has a poem in each issue, and other writers no less reckless serve to keep the interest going. You might find a sample copy worth a few spare stamps. Possibly.

THE TROUBLE ABOUT FASTING

is there's no place to do it.

Unless you're evolved far enough to find Nature alone a sufficient companion, guide, and inspiration. Your friends and relatives are all slaves of the Dinner-Bell; and they won't listen for a minute to your becoming emancipated right before their eyes. So you can't fast at home with any degree of satisfaction. Nor is a sojourn among strangers at all salutary—they won't understand and will gossip. Besides you're liable to get arrested if you take Sun Baths in the vicinity of so-called civilization—it isn't proper to go without clothes except at the sea-shore and on the stage.

The ideal spot for a long or short Fast has been discovered. It has plenty of woodland and hills; the clearest brook you ever drank from or dabbled in; places for Air Baths (parks separate for men and women); a mountain-view for twenty miles in all directions; the finest atmosphere and freshest breeze that the most ardent Breathing specialist could ask for; a soil surcharged with magnetism; enough space for all the solitude you require;—**and** people in charge who believe in Fasting and know how it should be done.

But suppose you'd rather eat—some folks would; quite sensible folks, too, in most respects. Then this is the place for you just as surely. Because the food is the best you ever tasted—nobody would imagine such a menu served at a Health Home. Business men come out from New York every Sunday just to revel in the country-ness of it all—and to rest for a fresh week's work. Massage, Baths, and other Naturopathic treatment if you want; or only quiet, reading and recreation.

There isn't a better place in the United States to spend all or part of your summer than at the **Naturopathic Health Home,** Butler, New Jersey. Yes, that's the spot—you won't ever forget it once you've been there. Open from May to November. Nights always cool—days just comfortable in the heart of the forest. Tents for those who like camping out— house accommodations for those who don't. Daily instruction and illustration of Natural Healing in its various phases—especially the Just System of Self-Healing. Fine opportunity for long walks and Nature study. Only 40 miles from New York and yet all the wildness of the deep recesses of the mountain-nook. People who come stay. Those who go come again. A single visit will do anybody good. That means you.

Circular sent freely. Write the New York office during winter months—address B. Lust, 124 East 59th Street, New York.

Important Notice.—The foregoing information should not be mistaken for advice. Nobody asks you to study Naturopathy, to believe in it, to investigate its claims. If you're wise you will; that's all. Those of us who have come close to Nature are bigger and better, healthier and happier, truer and saner, and surer of the eternal verities.

May you also triumph; aided equally by the solace of Nature, the power of Truth, and the inspiration of Love.